The Business of Maternity Care

by the same author

Complementary Therapies in Maternity Care
An Evidence-Based Approach
ISBN 978 1 84819 328 4
eISBN 978 0 85701 284 5

Aromatherapy in Midwifery Practice
ISBN 978 1 84819 288 1
eISBN 978 0 85701 235 7

The Business of Maternity Care

A GUIDE FOR MIDWIVES AND DOULAS SETTING UP IN PRIVATE PRACTICE

Denise Tiran

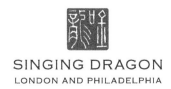

SINGING DRAGON
LONDON AND PHILADELPHIA

First published in 2019
by Singing Dragon, an imprint of
Jessica Kingsley Publishers
73 Collier Street
London N1 9BE, UK
and
400 Market Street, Suite 400
Philadelphia, PA 19106, USA

www.singingdragon.com

Library of Congress Cataloging in Publication Data
A CIP catalog record for this book is available from the Library of Congress

British Library Cataloguing in Publication Data
A CIP catalogue record for this book is available from the British Library

ISBN 978 1 84819 386 4
eISBN 978 0 85701 385 9

Printed and bound in Great Britain

As always, this book is dedicated to my wonderful son, Adam, currently living in our beloved South Africa and working in the African music industry. Adam has been of great help as his own experience in the commercial world and his greater understanding of technology and social media has kept me sane. I miss you.

Contents

Acknowledgements

I would like to thank my editor at Singing Dragon, Claire Wilson, for giving me the opportunity to write this new book and to share my own experiences of establishing and maintaining my business with others embarking on private maternity-related practice.

Huge thanks go to my friends and business colleagues, members of Expect, my businesswomen's support group, and to all the midwives and doulas who have offered information and advice. I would like to thank, in particular, Joanne Bell of Bell's Accountants for her help with financial issues. Thanks, too, to the midwives and doulas who contributed case studies to the book: Jan Bastard, Sarah Bryan, Eleanor Fowler, Dianne Garland, Samantha Jones, Cassie Marnoch, and Amanda Redford. Also, a big thanks to Samantha Jones for reading the manuscript for me, and for her insightful comments.

My brother, Mark Huckle, who is my co-director in Expectancy, has been helpful with many business issues, offering advice, information and thoughts on some of the thorny business, legal and financial matters that have arisen over the years. Thanks also to my sister-in-law, Judith, for a bed (and gin!) when I've been travelling in their area of the country.

The Purpose of this Book

Having spent over 25 years writing professionally, primarily on maternity complementary therapies, but also on midwifery in general, this book is a move away from my usual subject area and has been an interesting one to write. In many respects it has been easier, not least because, unlike my last book, *Complementary Therapies in Maternity Care: An Evidence-Based Approach* (2018), which had 70 pages of research references, this one has only a few! Conversely, it has been more difficult putting into words the lessons I have learned since going into business for myself and trying to decide what information you may need to help you along your own journey to starting your business.

With this book I hope to provide you with some practical tips to help you decide if you wish to set up your own practice and to avoid some of the mistakes that I, and many others before me, have made. I hope to give you sufficient information to understand the steps you need to take, the important professional, legal and financial issues you should address, and the ways in which you can market your business to build a successful future.

You will, of course, have your own ideas about what you want to do, and it is important to trust your instincts, but also to know when – and how – to ask for help. Setting up a business means you are entering a whole new world and having to learn a completely new subject area and its jargon. People often talk about 'working *on* the business, not working *in* it' – meaning that it is equally necessary to spend time learning about and attending to the business matters that help your practice to thrive, as well as keeping up-to-date on maternity issues and how they relate to your own profession – and then doing the work of the practice on a day-to-day basis. Starting a new business venture requires blood, sweat and tears – but I hope, by reading this book, you will forge ahead with your ideas with an organised approach that ensures your success. Good luck!

1

Introduction

My journey from midwife to businesswoman

I always wanted to be a midwife, from the age of 15, specifically a community midwife. Like many, I had experienced the usual teenage desire to become a nurse but, for some unknown reason, I focused on becoming a midwife although no one in my family knew anything about the profession. My decision might have had something to do with wanting the status of being a doctor but not achieving adequate A-level grades to study medicine. When I left school in the 1970s, the normal route to midwifery was through nursing, so my mother took me to the school careers convention to find out more. She had a momentary panic when I announced I was going to train as a nurse in the Queen Alexandra's Royal Army Nursing Corps (presumably she was worried in case there was a war). However, she managed to dissuade me, and eventually I gained a place to study nursing at the prestigious St Bartholomew's Hospital in the City of London.

I spent a frustrating three years studying to be a nurse, enjoying obstetrics (of course) and specialities such as the emergency department and theatre work. I hated, with a vengeance, the routines of medical and surgical ward work, and was petrified by the intensive care unit. I am sure I was never really a good nurse because my heart was not in it. Thankfully I was 'released' from nursing and commenced midwifery training in North London almost immediately. I returned to Bart's on qualifying and spent a pleasant few months working permanent night duty on the labour ward to consolidate my learning.

Unusually for the time, within a year of becoming a midwife, I was given the opportunity to take up a community-based post in Surrey, mainly practising midwifery, but with some district nursing included (unfortunately – too many elderly calloused feet to dress!). I enjoyed just over a year of having my own caseload, conducting home births and becoming known within the local area as 'the midwife'. I remember the father of one of the mothers commenting on the fact that I was not a typical district midwife because I was not 40, wearing a cap and riding a bike! I was just 24 years old, always threw my cap on the back seat of the car, and would have had difficulty completing my day's work on a bike as there were sometimes ten miles between visits.

Indeed, I quickly recognised that there was not sufficient mental stimulation from the work I was doing. This was not because I disliked community work – no, I loved it and still, almost 40 years later, I remain committed to community midwifery. However, working in a very rural area meant there was just not enough to do. I am sure today's midwives find that difficult to believe and perhaps wish they could say the same, given the 21st-century workload in the National Health Service (NHS) maternity services. After some deliberation, I decided to go into midwifery teaching and initially took a post as an obstetric tutor in Central London, teaching student nurses undertaking their mandatory four-week obstetrics placement. About a year later I moved to a small maternity unit in South East London, which was part of the then Greenwich and Bexley School of Midwifery. I was seconded to complete my Postgraduate Certificate in Education (PGCE) at the University of Surrey and returned to work in what had evolved into the School of Health at the University of Greenwich.

Once working in the higher education sector, numerous opportunities arise for lecturers to develop areas of interest and expertise. In the early 1980s, midwives were required to attend a one-week refresher course every five years, and tutors were allowed to attend one course that was not midwifery-specific but on a subject that could be applied to midwifery. I opted to attend a week-long course to qualify in massage. I returned to the university and started to include massage in my teaching of students and my care of women.

Following a very short break for maternity leave (a home birth), I then decided to attend what I thought was a reflexology course, but which turned out to be a specific German clinical style called reflex zone therapy, developed by a midwife, Hanne Marquardt. I was still breastfeeding my son at the time, and was amazed to experience increased lactation whilst on the course. The tutor explained that, during the previous day's practical work, my colleague had slightly over-stimulated the reflex zones for the pituitary gland on my feet. A passion was born! Reflex zone therapy became – and remains – my principal therapy, and I find it fascinating how it applies to pregnancy, birth and postnatal care. The following year I completed an aromatherapy qualification but, whilst the tutor was a lovely therapist, she was not a good teacher, and I was largely self-taught in terms of the theory.

Back at the University of Greenwich I had been asked to develop a short introductory post-registration module on complementary therapies for qualified nurses and midwives. The general public was increasingly interested in using 'alternative' medicine and the complementary professions were gradually formalising their pre-registration training courses and continuing education, as well as the services available, albeit almost entirely private at this stage. Whilst palliative care, particularly oncology, was the clinical field most fervently embracing complementary therapies, interest amongst pregnant women was also steadily rising. This was mainly because women wanted non-medical alternatives to deal with the many discomforts of pregnancy. Somewhat erroneously, they perceived complementary therapies as being safer than drugs because they are natural (a misconception that persists today). Suffice it to say that midwives and doctors were increasingly being asked about complementary therapies and natural remedies but were not sufficiently informed to be able to advise women appropriately. This short module eventually evolved into first, a Diploma of Higher Education and later, a full undergraduate Bachelor of Science Honours (BSc Hons) degree programme on complementary therapies, which I developed and managed for 14 years. I continued my own learning and completed a Master's degree in Health Research for which I investigated the safety of aromatherapy in pregnancy. In the complementary medicine field I studied herbal medicine, homeopathy and Bach flower remedies, learned how to use moxibustion for women with breech presentation and read voraciously on nutrition and other aspects of complementary medicine. I also completed a course in sexual counselling and, several years later, I trained in clinical hypnosis for childbirth and maternity acupuncture.

As part of the degree programme I set up a specialist clinic for pregnant women booked for birth at one of the maternity units in South East London. The unit served as a placement area for student midwives and the intention was to provide a teaching clinic for students on the BSc (Hons) Complementary Therapies, as well as for student and qualified midwives and occasionally doctors visiting from around the UK and from overseas. The clinic ran one day a week and over a ten-year period I treated around 6000 pregnant women. I gained enormous experience in using complementary therapies to treat physiological discomforts and specific problems in pregnancy, labour and the puerperium. I used an integrated approach in which I combined a range of complementary therapies with normal midwifery practice. I developed a particular interest in treating women suffering from nausea and vomiting, using complementary therapies and natural remedies combined with conventional strategies (see Tiran 2004).

During the time that I worked at the University of Greenwich, having written a couple of short review articles on complementary therapies for midwifery journals, I was asked to contribute a chapter on the subject to one of the main midwifery textbooks, *Mayes' Midwifery* (Sweet and Tiran 1990). Quite by chance, the editor mentioned that she was looking for someone to write a whole book on complementary therapies in pregnancy – and the rest is history, as they say. My first two books were published in the early 1990s, and several others followed over the next decade, together with dozens of papers for professional midwifery and complementary therapy journals and several chapters in midwifery and obstetric textbooks. I was also encouraged to engage in several research studies at the university, firmly cementing my place in becoming an authority on complementary therapies in pregnancy and childbirth. I stayed in mainstream midwifery and university teaching for almost 25 years.

I always say that I was in the right place at the right time insofar as developing the subject into a specialism in its own right, and I feel fortunate to have been the first midwife to become fully engaged in this field. My various publications informed the wider professional audience, and since then I have taught in many countries, notably in Japan, where I have been teaching pregnancy aromatherapy for almost 20 years. I have also been invited to speak at national and international conferences for midwives, doulas, antenatal teachers, obstetricians and complementary practitioners. More recently I am proud to have been honoured with the award of Fellowship of the Royal College of Midwives for my work in the field of midwifery complementary therapies.

However, for a long time, I had had the idea of working for myself, and eventually burn-out at the university led me to follow my dream. I started planning in 2003, whilst continuing to work four days a week, running the degree programme and managing home life with a four-year-old in between. As my plans progressed, I felt as if I was working 'eight days a week' in order to fulfil all my commitments. Finally, there came a point when I had to take the gigantic leap into the unknown world of the commercial sector. It was probably the scariest thing I have ever done. There is nothing like having to bring in an income to motivate you to succeed in a fledgling business.

Expectancy has now been running for 15 years, offering a unique range of accredited courses for midwives and doulas on different aspects of complementary therapies. For the first few years I did everything myself, with some help from a midwifery lecturer colleague who had a similar background to my own. Later, the administration became so unwieldy that I needed a virtual assistant, who has been with me ever since and is responsible for all the student administration. I have a team of freelance lecturers and we provide a whole range of study days, short courses and long programmes of study including the Diploma in Midwifery Complementary Therapies and the Certificate in Midwifery Acupuncture. Expectancy has evolved over the years and is the leading provider of specialist training on maternity complementary therapies. Scheduled courses are held in London but training is also delivered in maternity units, universities and colleges around the UK and overseas.

More recently I have added business mentoring and coaching for midwives and doulas wanting to move into private practice. I offer Business Masterclasses and a specific business training programme to help colleagues set up their practice and provide ongoing business support once their businesses are established. I have also diversified into providing help for other businesswomen through my new company, Expect Business Support, based in South East London. Expect offers a monthly problem-solving forum for women running their own businesses who want to be part of a membership-only, cohesive group in which they can discuss successes, failures and ongoing problems in a confidential setting. This is not specifically a networking group (see Chapter 5 on networking), but evolved from discussions with colleagues and friends who felt they wanted more than just the opportunity to meet new people and gain customers. It can be very lonely running your own business, and Expect offers a chance to get together on a regular basis and share issues that might be difficult to discuss with staff involved in one's own specific field.

Case study: Denise Tiran MSc RM PGCEA

expectancy

Expectancy (www.expectancy.co.uk) is an education company offering accredited courses for midwives on the safety and implementation of complementary therapies in pregnancy and childbirth. It is based in London and the South East, and is both national and international.

I formally set up Expectancy in 2003 (as a limited company registered with Companies House). I eventually left my post as Principal Lecturer (midwifery/complementary therapies) at the University of Greenwich and started trading in December 2004. My brother, a successful businessman, is my co-director, and together we put in £45,000 to get the company off the ground, which we were able to repay within two years. Initially, the intention was to offer clinical services to women in South East London as well as professional courses but, for a variety of reasons, the midwifery colleagues who had initially opted to join me withdrew, and this focused my attention solely on teaching.

Expectancy offers a range of short courses and study days, as well as a unique Diploma in Midwifery Complementary Therapies and a Certificate in Midwifery Acupuncture. Our scheduled courses are held in London and include aromatherapy, reflexology, massage, hypnosis, acupuncture, acupressure, moxibustion (for breech presentation), natural remedies and complementary therapies for post-dates pregnancy and for nausea and vomiting. I also provide on-site courses in NHS maternity units around the UK for midwives to introduce complementary therapies into their service provision, and for student midwives in universities, both in the UK and overseas. I have been teaching in Japan for almost 20 years but have also been invited to teach in Hong Kong, Malta, Italy, Iceland, Canada and Norway. I have recently negotiated a long-term contract to teach two or three times a year in various cities in China. Expectancy's annual income is over £100,000 and we have recently had to register for VAT (payable to HMRC once turnover exceeds £83,000 in any one year).

Your greatest achievements? I am proud to have been awarded a Fellowship of the Royal College of Midwives for my work in the specialist field of maternity complementary medicine (2018), as well as being highly commended in the Prince of Wales' Awards for Healthcare in London (2001) and winning the Complementary and Alternative Medicine award for services to education in 2011. In business terms, I think my greatest achievements must be keeping the business going through two economic recessions and being a runner-up in the Kent Women in Business Awards (2015).

Your biggest mistake? Advertising – in the early days I completely over-spent on advertising that was poorly focused and spread far too widely. This was mainly because we had not adequately delineated our target market and were trying to sell to too many different groups. Initially, I had a team of midwives who all practised different complementary therapies, and we were intending to offer services to pregnant women in the local area. At the same time I was trying to promote educational courses – for midwives, doulas, antenatal teachers and for complementary practitioners wanting to work with pregnant women. Needless to say there was a lot of wasted expenditure that did not bring in any real income.

How has your business evolved? Initially, I offered courses for midwives, doulas, antenatal teachers and complementary therapists, but I finally made a conscious decision to focus solely on providing courses for midwives and students (although I also teach maternity workers, therapists and medical practitioners when requested). In the last four years, in response to growing demand, I have set up a Licensed Consultancy scheme to help midwives wanting to work in private practice offering maternity-related services. The scheme includes training in the relevant complementary therapies as well as business training and clinical mentoring to set up and maintain the practice. As time goes on, I will need to start looking at succession planning so that others can take over the teaching and possibly buy the company once I am ready to retire (if ever!).

What is the best thing about working for yourself? Being in control of what you want to do and being able to make decisions about the business without the bureaucracy of a large organisation.

What causes you most difficulty in running your own business? Anything official: dealing with HMRC, completing the accounts, legal issues, etc. Never having enough time for myself – and the impact this has on my partner.

What advice would you give to a midwife/doula who is just setting out in the commercial world? Follow your dream but take time to plan, get help from experts and learn from your mistakes.

I have come a long way since those early days and made many mistakes along the way – more of that later. I have worked harder than ever before (and running a programme at the university was hard work), but I do not regret moving into the commercial world. I love working for myself and would not want to return to full-time employment, either within the health services or the higher education sector. I now want to be able to help others who are considering directing their maternity-related expertise and experience into private practice – hence this book. I hope it will provide a useful resource to get you started on your journey to self-employment and to running a successful business.

Trends in maternity care: justifying the move towards offering private services for expectant and new mothers

When I first became a midwife, life was much simpler. Indeed, midwifery in the late 1970s was not so very different from that portrayed in the television series *Call the Midwife* set in the early 1960s, in which the midwife was a respected pillar of society, and women and their families were compliant, deferred to authority and rarely challenged professional decisions. There were no mobile telephones, no internet or social media and few educational television programmes, so the knowledge of birth remained shrouded in mystery for many of the general public. Whilst some women worked, many did not. For the few who did work outside the home, the maternity benefits system encouraged them to stop working in the early third trimester and to rest and plan for the births of their babies and prepare for motherhood. The majority of women then stayed at home to care for their children, possibly for some years after giving birth.

Nowadays, many women expect to wait until their late thirties or even their forties before trying to conceive. This may be partly financially driven, but is also due to the change in women's roles and their desire to progress up the career ladder in the same way as men. For those who may once have found it difficult to conceive later in life, there are now medical advances to provide assisted conception. Once they are pregnant, women assume that they can continue to work until term, and are often frustrated when normal physiological discomforts affect their capacity to do so. They expect labour to start spontaneously, on the 'due date' (or possibly before), and that they will labour without pain relief or intervention – or conversely, with all the medication and technology that modern obstetrics has to offer. Afterwards, new mothers seem to think they will fit back into their pre-pregnancy jeans immediately, get back to work after six weeks, and that the baby will fit nicely into a convenient routine in which the baby wakes to feed four-hourly and sleeps in between. These somewhat unrealistic expectations contribute to immense emotional and social problems for women. Many have the disposable income to buy anything they want. However, they fail to appreciate that having a baby is something that cannot be controlled; nor can they buy their way out of all the problems or difficulties that may arise.

In addition, the maternity services in the UK have changed out of all recognition. In the late 1960s most babies were still being born at home, but in 1970 *The Peel Report* (DH 1970) advocated that all births should take place in hospital, a trend that largely continues today, despite a few valiant attempts to change this. As a result, there was much greater medical interference, leading to demands in the 1980s for improvements in the maternity services (MSAC 1982,

1984, 1985). In 1982 I even attended a rally on London's Hampstead Heath campaigning for a greater focus on natural birth. Later still, the *Changing Childbirth* report (DH 1993) proposed that the maternity services be based on 'choice, continuity and control' for women. More recently, the Better Births campaign (National Maternity Review 2016) again appealed for a change from interventionist obstetrics to a more physiological approach to birth. Having worked in and around the maternity services for so many years, I have seen the same problems come around several times – and still there is significant consumer dissatisfaction with the care that women receive during pregnancy and birth.

On the other hand, the demands put on the maternity services have also increased exponentially. We now have an annual UK birth rate of almost three-quarters of a million (ONS 2016) and a diverse multi-cultural society, with high levels of recently arrived immigrants in some areas, all with different attitudes to pregnancy and different needs. Huge burdens are put on all areas of healthcare with the changing pathological demands of the population, for example, those who are morbidly obese, with all the consequences of obesity, or who have other complex physical, psychological or social needs. For various reasons, the number of Caesarean sections is almost out of control, with an average of 25 per cent across the UK, but with some units having a rate of almost 35 per cent (Campbell and Duncan 2016; personal communications with midwives). Added to this are the political and economic implications for the health services, with reduced budgets having to fund increased demands. Low staffing levels are widespread across almost all maternity units in England, leading to midwives who are exhausted, burnt-out, demoralised and disillusioned. Furthermore, a large proportion of the midwifery and nursing workforce is approaching retirement age, with fewer young people entering the profession, a factor that will only compound the problems in the next few years (Merrifield 2017). Added to this is the introduction of university tuition fees for those commencing midwifery (and nursing) degrees, with an ensuing reduction in applications and take-up of training places (personal communications with colleagues in higher education). Despite a pledge from the government to increase midwifery training places (BBC News 2018) there remains a deficit in the availability of midwifery posts on qualifying, an almost uncontrollable workload and a stampede of departures from the NHS by midwives who no longer feel able to provide women-centred care.

Consequently, priorities within the maternity services, of necessity, focus on women with complex needs, meaning that those who can achieve a physiological birth are often deprived of the time and support that would contribute to a more satisfying experience. The advent of doulas in the UK in the 1990s has provided much-needed additional emotional, physical and informational support and advocacy for women, during and after the birth. A recent Cochrane review (Bohren *et al.* 2017) suggests that women who have the continued intrapartum attendance of a doula or midwife are more likely to labour spontaneously and are less likely to require analgesia or operative delivery. These women also achieve improved breastfeeding success and are less likely to develop postnatal depression. Women are increasingly choosing to appoint a doula to ensure that they are not left unsupported because busy NHS midwives are unable to stay with them throughout their labours (Fearn 2015).

This fear has also fuelled an increase in the number of women opting to give birth without professional assistance – commonly known as 'free birthing'. Many choose this option to avoid the inherent medicalisation of labour that occurs in hospital, others for its empowering effect on their birthing and parenting experiences, and some because of previous traumatic intrapartum incidents in hospital. Rather than relying on professional support, most of these women prefer to have the help and support of their partners, friends, family or others to keep them physically comfortable and emotionally in control. Indeed, the apparently increasing incidence of tocophobia may not actually be related to a fear of the labour and birth itself, but rather to a fear of the maternity services and the anticipated care (or perceived lack of care) that they may receive. It is known that peripartum post-traumatic stress disorder (PTSD) can impact on a mother's relationship with her baby and on future pregnancies (Schwab, Marth and Bergant 2012).

Furthermore, pregnant women and their partners now frequently seek alternative, or complementary, services to those generally offered by the NHS. The demise, in many maternity units, of traditional antenatal classes has deprived expectant parents of opportunities to meet like-minded couples and to learn about the impending birth and parenthood. The social expectation to become a 'perfect' parent has resulted in increased stress during pregnancy and after birth, leading many women to opt for relaxation therapies, such as massage, aromatherapy and reflexology. Isolation is also often a problem for new mothers who have built a career for many years and whose social contacts are primarily colleagues rather than other mothers in their local area. The provision of group activities may help to overcome or reduce this social isolation.

Demands on the NHS may mean that essential services incur delays or are inadequate. Expectant mothers with moderately severe but non-pathological discomforts of pregnancy are often fobbed off with false reassurance, unwanted medication – or nothing at all – yet would gladly pay to receive support and treatment, perhaps in their own home, from a private practitioner. Examples of this include women with prolonged, distressing non-pathological sickness or those with backache, sciatica and pelvic girdle pain who have perhaps a ten-week wait for an NHS physiotherapy appointment (personal observations). The availability of private maternity acupuncturists, hypnotherapists or manual complementary practitioners would enable those women with the means and motivation to pay to seek prompt treatment that would facilitate a return to a relatively normal day-to-day life. Sometimes, all that women desire is an opportunity for a prolonged discussion with a midwife or doula who can answer their myriad questions and alleviate their concerns, and many would pay for enhanced antenatal care provision.

Postnatal care in the community is now almost non-existent compared to 30 years ago. In many areas, a midwife or even a healthcare assistant visits the mother just twice in the first ten days after the baby's birth. Whilst many parents would not want a return to the twice-daily or daily visits from a community midwife, especially when no appointment time is specified, they do miss out on the support that many need to help them recover from the birth, adapt to parenthood and establish breastfeeding. Lactation support in particular would be a popular option amongst these women. Parents of babies awaiting frenulotomy for tongue-tie and who are intent on breastfeeding will often be prepared to pay for an independent practitioner to perform the necessary incision within 24 hours of birth rather than having to wait for three weeks for an NHS appointment, as is the case in some areas. Other services may be considered non-essential and are not normally available on the NHS for the majority, such as preconception care, yet good preparation for pregnancy can prevent or reduce some of the bio-psycho-social issues that can occur.

All of these factors combine to provide a market for midwives and doulas wanting to offer private maternity-related services. Many women have some disposable income and are prepared to pay for alternative options such as NCT, 'hypnobirthing', yoga or water-based exercise classes. Although health systems in other countries differ from the UK, pregnancy and childbirth appear, across the world, to be something for which women want the best, both for themselves and for their babies. A study of over 1800 women in Australia (Adams *et al.* 2017) found that, whilst the majority of women used publicly funded or health insurance-funded standard maternity services, many were prepared to pay for alternative sources of antenatal care, and almost 50 per cent accessed complementary medicine practitioners. Even in Zambia, women from rural areas with high-risk pregnancies are willing to contribute financially towards a stay in a residential maternity home in order to be closer to emergency services, should they be needed (Vian *et al.* 2017). This desire to pay for services does not only apply to families with sufficient disposable income to be able to afford luxuries: many women will opt to pay for services that enhance their overall satisfaction with and enjoyment of pregnancy and parenthood, in preference to purchasing something else they deem non-essential at this time in their lives.

Box 1.1 lists some possible areas of maternity-related care that you may wish to consider as possible services that could be offered to women via your private work. Box 1.2 gives some suggestions for non-clinical business services relating to maternity care that you may wish to provide, depending on your expertise and interests, training and insurance.

BOX 1.1: Maternity-related services for which women are prepared to pay

Antenatal services

- Preconception information, screening and advice
- Support and information for couples undergoing fertility treatment
- 'Welcome to pregnancy' consultations – similar to a booking appointment, with time to ask questions and discuss options
- Ultrasound scanning, interpretation and advice
- Enhanced antenatal care, over and above standard NHS care
- Advice and support on tests and investigations in pregnancy
- Additional fetal monitoring – 'listening in' and an opportunity for time with a midwife
- Pregnancy nutrition and dietary advice and support
- Advice on work, benefits, travel in pregnancy, etc.
- Maternity bra fittings, help with decision-making about infant feeding
- Antenatal classes in preparation for birth, including 'hypnobirthing' and relaxation sessions
- Massage workshops to teach couples how to use massage in labour
- Relaxation therapies for pregnancy – massage, aromatherapy, reflexology, shiatsu
- Acupuncture for sickness, backache, sciatica, constipation, etc.
- Specialist home visiting/intravenous supplementation for women with severe nausea and vomiting/hyperemesis gravidarum
- Exercise classes/one-to-one for pregnancy – Pilates, yoga, water-based activities
- Moxibustion for breech presentation
- Advice on complementary therapies and natural remedies in pregnancy, labour, postnatally
- Clinical hypnosis or counselling for tocophobia, needle phobia, etc.
- Help to stop smoking – hypnosis, counselling, relaxation therapies, conventional methods
- Maternity advocacy – accompanying women to antenatal appointments

- Support for women with specific psychological conditions – previous birth trauma, pre-existing depression or current/previous antenatal mental health issues

- Support for those with specific social conditions – domestic abuse, work issues, language difficulties

- Advice, information and care for women with multiple pregnancy, pre-eclampsia, diabetes and other medical or obstetric conditions

Birth-related services

- One-to-one preparation for birth and parenthood

- Specialist support for women approaching elective Caesarean section

- Advice and information on pain relief in labour – conventional and complementary

- Pre-birth acupressure and 'natural' induction of labour (see 'Case study: Samantha Jones', page 191)

- Full midwifery birth services (subject to indemnity insurance)

- Doula support in labour

- Complementary therapies for labour – pain relief, aiding progress in labour

- Placental encapsulation

Postnatal services

- Postnatal midwifery care to supplement standard NHS provision

- Postnatal doula care (see 'Case study: Eleanor Fowler', page 165)

- Postnatal support groups

- Lactation support

- Family planning and spacing advice

- Labour and birth reflection/'debriefing'

- Counselling, hypnosis or neurolinguistic programming (NLP) for postnatal mental health issues (see 'Case study: Cassie Marnoch', page 72)

- After-care for women who have had a Caesarean section

- Bereavement support – stillbirth, miscarriage, termination, loss of partner, mother, etc.

- Specialist pre- and post-birth consultations for partners

- Postnatal weight loss consultancy
- Cervical smears
- Private health visiting

Neonatal services

- Crying baby support
- Repeat examination of the new-born with time for in-depth discussion
- Frenulotomy and follow-up breastfeeding assistance
- Advice on baby care, weaning, immunisations, etc.
- Baby massage/teaching parents how to use baby massage
- Support for parents with a baby in special or intensive care unit
- Support for families with a baby born with physical disability, medical or genetic condition
- Sessions to teach parents basic first aid for their babies

BOX 1.2: Other, non-clinical, services you could offer in a freelance capacity

- Expert witness work (see 'Case study: Dianne Garland', page 92)
- Consultancy work for NHS trusts and private organisations – perhaps being involved in organisational change management or acting as an advisor for the Care Quality Commission (CQC)
- Lecturing to professionals if you have a teaching qualification and are a specialist in a particular field (see 'Case study: Denise Tiran', page 18)
- Advisory services to midwifery units or non-governmental organisations (NGOs) overseas
- Writing for publication – such as for a parenting magazine, or writing policy documents for NHS trusts and independent organisations
- Contracting with an insurance company to offer telemedicine consultations (usually requires nursing qualification as well as midwifery) or working in a triage situation for a charity or other organisation

- Undertaking short-term research projects for varying organisations

- Developing products such as aromatherapy oil blends for pregnant and newly birthed mothers (see 'Case study: Jan Bastard', page 53) or equipment such as the CUB birthing aid that was developed by a midwife,[1] or developing mobile telephone applications for pregnant women

Why 'the business of maternity care'?

The concept of the NHS, founded in 1948, in which healthcare was made available free at the point of access for everyone, was a social and political triumph and has served its purpose well for many decades. Unfortunately, it has become increasingly difficult to uphold these principles in more recent years as the effects of a growing and ageing population, changing demographics, medical advances and technological progress have led to ever-increasing financial burdens. Setting budgets for the NHS is largely dependent on political opinion and societal factors, with 78 per cent of the public now consistently rating healthcare spending as a top priority (Anadaciva 2017). However, irrespective of one's own political beliefs, the general public is beginning to realise that NHS resources are not infinite and that governments need to allocate national budgets across all publicly funded services, including not only health and social care, but also education, the emergency services, local council funding and more.

Unfortunately, the legacy of the NHS has generated a nation that has traditionally expected to receive *all* services free of charge. The funding of public budgets through taxation and National Insurance contributions, usually deducted from salaries at source, is a contentious subject, but many people fail to understand fully that they are, in fact, paying for their healthcare, albeit involuntarily and heavily subsidised. Further, a somewhat paternalistic system seems to obviate any real need for individuals to take responsibility for one's own health, engendering a notion that people can indulge in harmful behaviours and yet expect to be treated for their consequences.

---

1   www.cub-support.com

This lack of awareness extends to the 1.5 million people employed by an unwieldy NHS (Gerada 2014) in which individual clinical staff have no real obligation to manage local budgets. Most have no concept of the cost of specific tests and investigations, procedures or care provision. It has been suggested that computerised ordering and replenishment systems could reduce wastage due to over-ordering (Gbadamosi 2015) and engender considerable cost savings (Moore 2017), with individual staff becoming more aware of – and more accountable for – the equipment they are using. This is standard practice in private hospitals, where every single item is recorded, from major surgical procedures down to the smallest gauze swab or incontinence pad. If this practice was introduced into NHS care, there would doubtless be a reduction in monies wasted. Indeed, there is an urgent need to include an introduction to the funding and costs of healthcare in the educational programmes preparing all healthcare professionals – midwives, doctors, nurses, physiotherapists, etc.

Midwives, doulas, doctors and other maternity professionals are usually unaware of the costs of antenatal, intrapartum, postnatal and neonatal care. To many NHS employees, 'money' is a subject best disregarded as it conflicts with their personal philosophy of free healthcare. Yet, as a nation, as professionals providing care and as responsible members of society, we can no longer ignore the fact that healthcare is big business. Everything must be paid for and therefore everything must be costed prior to use. Passing the onus to individuals to save money in their own practice so that limited funds can be prioritised may enable greater allocation of monies to those areas or those people who really need them. This concept does not have to be at odds with the absolute need for safe practice, but could, in fact, free up funds to enhance safety.

Somewhat cynically, one of the strongest arguments for the contemporary focus on a return to physiological birth appears to be the need to save money in addition to the desire to avoid expensive litigation. The cost of NHS antenatal care, physiological birth and postnatal care is now estimated at £2790 per birth, with care in labour costing around £750 (2015 National Tariff System). If complications occur, this could increase to £5000, with the price of a Caesarean section being approximately £1700 (2015 National Tariff System).

In the private sector, these costs rise to £2000 for a physiological birth and up to £7000 if there are complications, whilst an epidural anaesthetic is about £1395, an ultrasound scan costs at least £300 and a neonatal examination is £250 (Mulroy 2017).

Much has been written in recent years about the insidious privatisation of the NHS, particularly since the Health and Social Care Act 2012 was passed. However, private companies have always provided drugs, equipment, catering, cleaning, transport and portering services to the NHS. The NHS purchases nursing and midwifery pre-registration education from the higher education sector, and some post-registration training is provided by commercial organisations such as my own company, Expectancy. However, non-NHS provision of clinical services is more controversial, despite the fact that dentistry, optometry and pharmacy have been provided by the private sector for many years. In addition, most general medical practices are legally set up as private partnerships. Increasingly, the NHS is moving towards 'outsourcing', in other words, giving contracts to private companies to run NHS services. This market-based approach is considered to increase competition so that resources purchased can be cost-effective and also serve as a means of expanding choice for patients. Some of this is achieved through the *Any Qualified Provider* (AQP) scheme (see Chapter 2), whilst other services are provided by social enterprises, charitable organisations and community interest companies. A King's Fund report (2015) identified that approximately £10 billion of the total £113 billion NHS budget was spent on care from non-NHS providers (not including dentistry, pharmaceutical and general practice services).

The Health and Social Care Act makes it mandatory for Clinical Commissioning Groups (CCGs) to put services out to competitive tender if they can potentially be provided from outside the NHS. Between 2010 and 2015 non-NHS providers were responsible for 86 per cent of pharmacy services, 83 per cent of patient transport facilities, 76 per cent of diagnostic services, 69 per cent of general practitioner (GP)/out-of-hours services, 45 per cent of community health services and 25 per cent of mental health services (Patients4NHS 2018).

There is also a move towards the NHS charging for some services in addition to prescriptions, dental care and eye tests (although these are heavily subsidised). In maternity care, some units charge for antenatal or 'hypnobirthing' classes, introduction to water birth sessions and, occasionally, complementary therapy services such as acupuncture (personal communications with midwives and managers). Some of these services are provided by NHS midwives employed within the maternity unit, or by midwives and antenatal teachers working in a private capacity in their own time; others are provided by appropriately trained independent practitioners who have contracted their services to the NHS. The services that midwifery managers are prepared to contract out are often deemed to be 'non-essential', allowing allocation of limited NHS resources to priority areas such as the care of women with complex physical, mental or social needs. However, the fact that many women choose to pay for these services implies that there is a need to provide them in some form.

The advent of a Personal Maternity Care Budget (PMCB), being trialled at the time of writing, aims to empower women and increase their choices for care during pregnancy, birth and the puerperium. It is thought that it may also offer a means of utilising providers from within and without the NHS. There will be no direct payment of monies, but each woman will be allocated a sum of money from which she is able to make choices, whilst remaining flexible enough to account for complications arising or the need for an alternative maternity care pathway. For women to take advantage of services provided by non-NHS organisations private practitioners, including independent midwives, doulas, complementary therapists and antenatal teachers, will need to have a contract with the local CCG within one of the pioneering areas where the woman lives.[2] Women will only be able to use their PMCBs to access maternity services commissioned by their CCGs, and will not be able to use them to help purchase private maternity care.[3]

---

2   See www.england.nhs.uk/commissioning

3   www.england.nhs.uk/mat-transformation/mat-pioneers/questions-and-answers-about-maternity-pioneers/personal-maternity-care-budgets-pmcbs

Making the decision to work for yourself

Midwives working in the NHS are increasingly disillusioned with the care they are able to provide for women (personal discussions with numerous midwives on courses, at conferences, by telephone and on social media). Many feel that the demands of midwifery practice today do not meet the ideals that caused them to enter the profession in the first place. The workload is phenomenal, with a risk-averse dependence on physio-pathological monitoring and the prevention or management of complications. Midwives have little time or energy to provide the psycho-emotional and social support that is so much a part of holistic maternity care. Long shifts leave them exhausted, although this does mean that they have more days off in the week. However unrealistic and unhealthy, shift patterns in which midwives are expected to transfer from day to night duty and back again within a week mean that they spend off-duty time recovering and resting, which may have a potentially deleterious effect on their health and family life. Older midwives may struggle to cope with the physical demands of the work, and many opt for retirement earlier than they might otherwise have done, further depleting the dwindling workforce.

As a result, midwives are increasingly choosing to set up in private practice or to establish other businesses aimed at enhancing women's experiences of pregnancy, birth and early parenthood. Many midwives telephone me to discuss working for themselves, and what started as a dribble of enquiries a couple of years ago is fast turning into a deluge. Many want to offer some private services whilst continuing to work part time within the NHS or for one of the emerging private companies that provide full maternity services. Some midwives are keen to work as doulas so that they can be 'with woman' without the litigation-conscious bureaucracy of the NHS or the legal responsibility of conducting births on their own accountability.

There is also, of course, a market for those who are not midwives but who actively choose to work as doulas. Often these women (and sometimes, men) have worked in jobs that have become mundane and unfulfilling and, despite potentially taking a reduction in income, become committed to working in a caring role. Some doulas come to the role as a result of their own positive birth experience and then wish to help others to achieve that for themselves. Alternatively, those who have had a negative birth experience may be motivated to help others avoid similar circumstances. Many doulas might have considered training to become a midwife, but for various reasons decide against it, preferring to offer services for pregnant and childbearing women in a manner of their choosing.

It is important to decide if going into business is for you and why you are considering it. Are you running away from a situation that may have become intolerable, or towards an ideal? If you are a midwife simply trying to get away from a difficult work environment, this may not be the best motivation for working for yourself; it may set you up to fail and should not be the only driving force behind your decision, although it may be a trigger to the overall process. Similarly, for doulas, whilst personal experience can be valuable in formulating your own opinions about what *you* would choose for maternity care, it is important not to permit your own feelings to colour your ability to decide objectively about going into business. On the other hand, if you decide that you want to make a difference, you want to help families to achieve a satisfying pregnancy and birth experience that they are unable or less likely to achieve from merely receiving standard NHS maternity care, this will present an outcome for which you can aim.

It is useful to spend some time really working out what you want to do, why you want to do it and what you have to offer, to help get your thoughts in order. Your decisions will depend on your personal and family circumstances, your age, experience, qualifications and your personal and professional philosophy. Activity 1.1 poses some questions to start this process. You do not have to answer all the questions, and some may take longer to mull over than others. Some questions may seem similar to others but sometimes looking at the issue again may give you a different perspective. Take time to complete this activity, noting down your thoughts and making comments, perhaps returning to them every couple of days so you can reflect further on your intended move into your own business.

🐾 ACTIVITY 1.1: Making the decision to set up in your own business (1)

— *Why* do you want to set up a private practice or work outside mainstream maternity care? Try to define *precisely why* you are thinking about working for yourself and what you want from the work you do. What personal vision do you have for yourself and what motivates you to do your 'own thing'? What are the long-term plans for your career and your personal life, and how might these affect, or be affected by, your plans to work in your own business? In other words, where do you see yourself in five, ten or even fifteen years' time?

— *What exactly* do you want from your professional working life? What is important to you about your work — and does this produce an acceptable work–life balance for you? What are the most important aspects of your current work that give you job satisfaction? What factors are important to you so that you enjoy your work? What motivates you to do a good job? How often do you go home at the end of a working day satisfied with what you have achieved?

- *Where* do you feel most comfortable working? This question might be interpreted in terms of geographical location, clinical environment, institution, peripatetic or home-based work. Try to analyse the reasons for your answers.

- *When* do you most like working? This may be based on whether you are a 'morning' or 'evening' person or whether you prefer summer or winter. It may relate to the period of the childbearing year that you find most interesting and the time at which you most enjoy working with women – pregnant, labouring or newly birthed.

- *Who* do you like working with most? Again, this could refer to the women for whom you most enjoy caring: antenatal, intrapartum or postnatal women or their babies and other family members or specific client groups such as women with medical conditions or social situations. You also need to think about the colleagues with whom you like working, and why this may be so. Are there any people (clients/colleagues) you feel are the most demanding?

— *How* do you want to work? Do you want to leave your current employment completely/permanently or do you want to work part time in your current work and part time in your own business? Do you see your business venture as a long-term/part-time/small or huge project?

— How much money do you want/need to earn? What could you not live without? What are your attitudes towards money and wealth? Indeed, how would you define 'wealth' in terms that are important to you?

✎ ACTIVITY 1.2: Making the decision to set up in your own business (2)

Now, compile two lists of what, for you, are the positive and negative aspects of setting out on your own. These may include professional issues (e.g., leaving the NHS completely means you have to pay for your own continuing professional development (CPD)), personal (e.g., able to manage time and work when it fits in with your family), financial or other factors that you feel are important or relevant to your life. You may also want to consider here your personal philosophy, the issues that drive you and the thoughts you have had whilst undertaking Activity 1.1.

Positive	Negative

Making the decision to work for yourself is incredibly liberating. Somehow things fall into place and the frustrations and trials and tribulations of your existing job become inconsequential. You feel empowered simply by making the initial decision and later, by the realisation that you can do things *your* way without recourse to innumerable committee meetings or the need to adhere to pedantic policies or directives. This is the opportunity of a lifetime, and once you have made that decision, it heralds an exciting time in your life.

It is also terrifying! For midwives in particular, the move from the protected environment of the NHS to the aggressive commercial world is more daunting than anything you will have encountered as a midwife. Even for doulas who may previously have been employed in the commercial sector, taking ultimate responsibility for making your own business a success can be equally intimidating. However, this can be a trigger to ensuring that you plan well in order to avoid the numerous pitfalls that come with moving into business. A little adrenaline goes a long way towards making your business a success.

Have you got what it takes?

You may ask yourself whether you possess the most appropriate skills and personal characteristics to go into business. Not everyone has the right frame of mind to go it alone, but the fact that you are considering private practice suggests that you are at least partway there. There is a lot to learn about how to set up, market and run a business, things you will probably have known very little about as an employee, especially working in a large bureaucratic organisation such as the NHS. You need more than just an ambition and the drive to achieve it. However, you will be surprised to identify the skills you have gained from your experience as a midwife or doula that can be applied to running a private practice and developing your own business. Indeed, training to become and then working as a midwife or doula facilitates the development of a wide range of transferable skills that will stand you in good stead for your business.

Personal attributes needed for a successful business
Passion and motivation

Once you decide to set up your own practice, you will spend all your time living and breathing it, certainly until it is well established. If you are not passionate at the start of the process you will find it difficult to continue when things get tough (and they will). Before making a final decision about setting up in business, work out exactly what factors drive you and whether these provide you with the ultimate justification for working for yourself. Is it because you feel passionate about helping women to achieve the birth they want? Is it the desire to make money? Do you want greater control over your working life, perhaps enjoying leading and motivating others? Be honest with yourself about this – it may help to talk this over with a partner or friend who knows you well and with whom you feel comfortable in sharing your innermost thoughts about your professional and personal life. If you can channel your passion and aim for your goals, however difficult that may seem at this time, you are halfway towards succeeding.

Self-belief and self-confidence

You must believe in yourself and the services you intend to provide – if you do not believe in your abilities and in what you are offering, neither will your potential clients. You may feel lacking in confidence in relation to the business skills and knowledge you need, but one of the first lessons to learn is not to under-estimate yourself and what you have to offer. If you have been in clinical practice for some years you will have gained a wealth of experience working with women before, during and after childbirth, and they will view you as an expert on the subject. In addition, being able to remain optimistic will ensure that you can overcome or minimise many of the challenges that will undoubtedly face you along the way. You need to be able to sell yourself well so that clients will see the value of receiving from *you* the services for which they wish to pay.

Professionalism

Your training and experience has focused on behaving in a professional manner; registration with a national regulatory body such as the Nursing and Midwifery Council (NMC) or Doula UK requires you to act professionally at all times (see also Chapter 3 on professional issues). Maintaining that professionalism when working for yourself will be fundamental to the success of your business. Women will consult you because they trust you and believe that you can care for them appropriately and safely. A professional demeanour and way of working will enhance your credibility and help you to develop your own 'brand', and may make the difference between a potential client choosing your services or going elsewhere.

Objectivity

You need to remain objective. Of course, your business is personal to you, but if something goes wrong you must be able to stand back and reflect on the issue without taking it personally – it is business and is not a reflection on you.

Flexibility

Even if you are the most well-organised person, unexpected issues do occasionally arise and you need to be adaptable enough to cope with them. Be prepared to embrace change and see it as a positive challenge rather than as a negative inconvenience. One of my own recent concerns was the need to register with Her Majesty's Revenue & Customs (HMRC) for Value Added Tax (VAT). It seemed an inordinately complex undertaking to revise the accounting system in line with HMRC requirements, coupled with the threat of HMRC fines for late filing. It was only when an accountant colleague suggested that having to register for VAT was a positive factor in the business because it meant I was earning more that I took it on board and saw it in a more optimistic light.

Energy

Setting up and running a business is a marathon, not a sprint. It can also be very tiring, especially when you become stressed when things go wrong or need immediate action. Starting slowly and building up your business gradually will ensure you are more successful but will also enable you to pace yourself. Personality A-type people are generally more likely to make the move into running their own businesses, but the vital issue here is that you possess both the physical and mental energy to stay the course. You must look after yourself and prioritise the commercial, professional and personal demands in your life so that you do not become exhausted and even burnt-out. If you do not have the energy at the start, you will be less likely to succeed and grow your business. You need to be proactive, taking the initiative to move forward, and be assertive in achieving your dreams.

Knowing your limitations

You cannot be good at everything. Nobody is capable of fulfilling all the tasks or aspects of business management, and it is essential to ask for help before you find yourself struggling. It is better to pay someone to do something well for you than to become stressed in trying to complete the task – and then doing it poorly.

Support of your family and friends

It is vital that your family and friends support you in your new venture, even though they will probably not be actively involved in it. Discuss your plans with your partner or closest friend. Consider the impact of long hours spent focusing your attention on your business, especially in the early days. How will you achieve an acceptable work–life balance? Can you organise your business so that it fits in with family commitments such as school events, caring for an elderly relative or taking holidays at times that suit other family members?

One of the downsides of my own business is the time that I spend away from home, both around the UK and increasingly frequently, overseas. However, my partner and I have evolved a system that suits us both and, wherever possible, he will accompany me, something that will probably become more commonplace once he retires. Conversely, we each get time to ourselves, which is healthy for the relationship. Also, as my two best friends have moved away from London I see much less of them now, but we can often arrange to meet when I am teaching in their areas.

Professional skills needed for a successful maternity-related private practice

Expertise and experience in your specific field of work

Whilst it can be exciting as a newly qualified midwife to consider working for yourself, it is essential that you have gained sufficient experience of midwifery, the maternity services and the context in which care is provided for women in order to sustain a service for which women are prepared to pay. You must be skilled in the specific consultations you intend to provide, with appropriate qualifications and an ability to apply principles to practice. For doulas, it is a little different because your training will, to a certain extent, have prepared you for working for yourself from the point of completing your course. However, whether you are a doula or a midwife, it is important to be confident in your practice in order to develop your expertise because you will need to spend some of your time and energy on dealing with the business issues rather than on the professional aspects of your work.

If we use the analogy of learning to drive, lessons taken before you pass your test teach you the basics so that you know how to drive without accidents or causing problems to your vehicle. Once you have your licence, you consolidate these skills until you reach a point where you can drive competently and confidently without constantly having to look at the gears or thinking about the pedals. Now you can become competent in other aspects of driving, such as looking for directions, travelling in the dark or re-setting the satellite navigation system. In business, your primary profession (midwife or doula) can be likened to learning the initial skills of driving, whilst the development of the more sophisticated skills after passing the test relates to learning how to run your business. You need to be able to practise your 'day job' without really thinking about it so that you can concentrate on learning about finances, marketing and all the other aspects of being self-employed.

Leadership skills

You must feel confident in leading yourself and others, managing teams if you intend to take on staff and leading by example. There are many different types of leader and you should take time to appreciate the category into which you fit. Even if you work in sole practice, some aspects of standard midwifery, such as ward or department management, can be applied to the business environment. You may also have been involved in facilitating meetings and committees outside your work, such as in the Parent-Teacher Association (PTA), which will have developed your leadership, communication and negotiating skills.

Communication skills

As a midwife or doula you will already have developed refined listening and inter-personal skills when dealing with women and their families, as well as with your colleagues; these should be second nature to the way you work. If you are providing services because you feel passionate about women's experiences, you will want to treat each woman/family as an individual. People pay for – and expect – a good service, and it will be one of the things that sets you apart from others providing similar services. Good service in the caring professions implies not only safe practice, but also attending to those aspects that are sadly lacking in an over-pressurised NHS service. Women want time to talk, they need you to listen to them and they will pay to see someone who is empathetic to their needs but who can also be objective about what is required to help them. Similarly, if you are intending to employ other people, whether it is colleagues providing the same services as yourself, or perhaps receptionists and cleaners in a clinic, you require good people management skills to ensure a cohesive team.

In business, communication skills must be sophisticated, whether verbal, written or non-verbal (body posture etc.). The written word can sometimes be misinterpreted and it is vital to choose the right words, whether this is in emails, social media or correspondence. Communicating who you are and what you represent is also seen in the way you present yourself, how you speak, look, dress and behave. You may need to develop public speaking skills in order to disseminate your message to a wide audience, but this also requires you to know your subject inside-out and to present it with competence and confidence.

Negotiation skills

Working with others, whether in your own company or purchasing services from other companies (e.g., accountancy, legal advice) also requires you to be able to negotiate diplomatically but assertively. Most midwives, and many doulas, will have had experience of negotiating at some level within their work, with managers, junior staff and students and with women and their families. Some may have been involved in strategic-level committees and the development of service provision. However, dealing with people in a commercial environment can initially be daunting until you become familiar with the subject matter of the negotiation, whilst continuing to be guided by the experts to whom you have turned for professional advice. For example, if you are negotiating the design of a website, make sure you agree a fee and set a date for the first draft and for completion. Do not be intimidated by your business contacts or coerced into spending more money than you feel you can manage or is appropriate; ask for quotes from at least three companies to get a feel for the approximate price range – and be prepared to say 'no'.

Organisational and planning skills

This includes setting goals, right from the start, and working out ways to achieve them. Planning is key to any business and it is important not to become so enthusiastic early on that you forge ahead with a poorly planned idea that will appear amateurish to potential clients. You must be able to manage your time well including setting aside some time for yourself. As a community midwife or a doula with several clients, you will have achieved an organised way of working so that you complete the work within an appropriate time frame. Developing systems and processes to enable you to organise your business, clients, staff and other people with whom you communicate is also essential.

IT skills

You must have a good degree of literacy in relation to information technology (IT). If you do not know how to install and use basic Microsoft packages, how to create presentations, use spread sheets, desktop publishing software, presentation software or systems such as accounting software, it is probably money well spent to find someone to teach you. It may be worth contacting your local further education department or even local business organisations to see what workshops and courses are available in your area. You must also be competent at dealing with emails in a professional manner, using a professional business signature. Unfortunately, unless you intend to establish a large business, you will also need to be able to identify and deal with problems that may arise with hardware, software and other equipment such as printers – there is no IT department to call on in your own small business.

Numeracy and literacy skills

You must be good at dealing with numbers in order to manage your finances. Midwives are required to calculate drug dosages and, at a senior level, to manage budgets and resources, and those intending to work as doulas may already have had to deal with financial affairs within previous jobs. At the very least you will probably have to deal on a regular basis with family finances. You can employ or contract someone to help you with your business accounts, but you must be able to deal with the income and outgoings (cash flow) in order to make a living and avoid unapproved debt. Similarly, you need to be able to present written communications to your prospective clients, business contacts and any staff you employ. If this is not your strong point, get help with proofreading before sending anything to clients, other professionals, business contacts or for printing.

Clerical skills

You must be able to perform basic clerical and administrative tasks, organise and manage your records and reports and design forms and means of correspondence to be used in your business. You should be able to take accurate, concise minutes at any meetings you arrange and keep track of decisions and actions required – if you have been a member of any committee, such as the local residents' association, this will help you to refine these skills. In any case, your need to maintain clinical records diligently, contemporaneously and comprehensively will stand you in good stead here.

Marketing and sales skills

This can be one of the most difficult areas for midwives and doulas whose primary objective is in caring for their clients. You need to understand what your clients actually want – and run the business for them. You will need to overcome the natural altruistic reservations about pricing that many caring professionals can experience – you are in business to make money, even though it may be offering services about which you are passionate (see Chapter 4 on financial issues and Chapter 5 on sales and marketing).

Now have a go at completing Activities 1.3 and 1.4 to identify your personal strengths and weaknesses.

⚡ ACTIVITY 1.3: Identifying your personal strengths and weaknesses (1)

—   Compile a list of your personal characteristics and the professional skills you currently employ in your work, using the ones discussed above as a starting point. It can be difficult to identify your 'good points' as many of us are inclined to be naturally modest. Try imagining if someone else was asked to define your strengths – what would they say?

—   Make a list of all the skills you have acquired in your previous work situations, both in maternity care-related work and from other jobs. This might include numeracy, from medicines management, negotiating skills in meetings or in dealing with anxious and perhaps argumentative relatives or attention to detail as a result of maintaining comprehensive records. You might also like to consider the skills you have gained in your personal life – for example, being a parent requires you to develop planning, budgeting, negotiation and communication skills.

—   What do you consider to be your *specific* strengths in the workplace? What experiences from other workplaces are useful in your current job? What are you most proud of having achieved in your professional life? If you are in a senior position in your current post, why do you think you were appointed? What is the best feedback you have ever received from a client or colleague at work? If you were asked to conduct your own annual appraisal, on which aspects would you focus?

—   Now try to list the things that cause you difficulty, the things you do not like doing and those that you would like to improve on. In your current work what do you consider to be your biggest challenge? What is the most demanding aspect of your working day? In which areas of your work do you feel you need to improve? In what situations do you ask for help? How do you feel when you are outside your comfort zone? What are you like in times of stress in the workplace? Try not to be too hard on yourself, but see this as a positive exercise to help you acknowledge where you may need to ask for, and probably to pay for, outside help in setting up your business.

ACTIVITY 1.4: Identifying your personal strengths and weaknesses (2)

In a more abstract way, try also to think about who you are, what motivates you and how you deal with things that occur in your professional and personal life.

— With which of your personal qualities are you most satisfied?

— How do you get on with people in general? What kind of first impression do you think you make?

— What issues in society interest you most? What incidents in your life have changed you, and how?

— What has been the greatest achievement in your personal life? What would you tell someone about yourself that would surprise them?

— What things upset you and what happens when you get upset? What mistakes have you made that you will never forget, and how did you deal with these and learn from them?

Are there any gaps you need to address by obtaining additional training or experience? This may be in terms of your professional role, but almost certainly will also include the need to develop good business skills.

How is working for yourself different from being employed?

Working in your own business can be exciting, interesting, stimulating, motivating and bring you a great sense of achievement and satisfaction. It can also be intimidating, worrying, lonely, exhausting and sometimes almost overwhelming. You need to consider, before you embark on the planning stage, whether you are able to deal with the 'downs' as well as the 'ups' and indeed, whether you have the energy, tenacity, motivation and drive to continue. When you have given some thought to both the advantages and disadvantages of working for yourself, you can then think more reflectively about whether or not this new venture is for you. Table 1.1 highlights some of the advantages and disadvantages of working for yourself.

Table 1.1: Advantages and disadvantages of working for yourself

ADVANTAGES	DISADVANTAGES
Personal autonomy	
You choose how the business operates, how, where and when you work and the services you wish to provide You can work towards having a better work–life balance (eventually) You can pursue your passion, build a reputation, develop a personal brand and inspire others	You are completely accountable for your actions, both from a professional and a business (financial, legal) perspective You may work more hours than ever before, especially at the outset You may be at risk of allowing your passion to overrule your business objectivity
Business management	
You determine the culture of your business Working for yourself enables you to avoid the bureaucracy of large organisations You can delegate boring tasks to others You have the potential to deviate into other ventures	It can be difficult to get the right balance between working enough to earn money and not taking on too much work You need the tenacity to follow things through before moving on to new initiatives

Communication	
You will be able to meet new people and develop a network of business colleagues whose skills complement your own You can use all means of communication and social media, focusing on those that you prefer or with which you are most familiar	Working for yourself can be lonely and isolating and it can be difficult to keep up-to-date with professional issues Running your own business can also impact on your family communication, relationships and friendships
Financial aspects	
This is your opportunity to invest in yourself A successful business will ultimately give you financial independence There may be some tax benefits to being self-employed Once you are established, you will have more job stability with no risk of being made redundant	You must earn enough for your financial needs Cash flow can be a problem There may be no government financial benefits – maternity leave, sick pay, holiday pay Personal and business financial security may be difficult to maintain

Case study: Jan Bastard BSc (Hons), RN, RM, IAIM

Motherlylove (www.motherlylove.co.uk), an international company selling natural skincare products for pregnancy.

I began planning my business in 2011 and launched the company in 2012. Having consciously retired from clinical midwifery when we moved to East Anglia, I still wanted to do something to help the health and wellbeing of women and babies. I had worked as a midwife and nurse in the UK and in Africa for over 40 years, and had completed the BSc (Hons) in Complementary Therapies at the University of Greenwich with Denise Tiran; I later went on to qualify as an aromatherapist. Our paper, 'Aromatherapy and massage for antenatal anxiety, its effect on the fetus', published in the *Complementary Therapies in Clinical Practice* journal (Bastard and Tiran 2009, first published 2006), emphasised the science behind the use of aromatherapy in pregnancy and childbirth.

I wanted to offer a range of skincare products and was fortunate to be able to develop these without needing to find finance. The products are fully tested for purity and quality (never on animals), vegan-friendly, and free of preservatives, fragrances, colourings and other harmful chemicals often used in beauty care products. They are approved by the Aromatherapy Trade Council (ATC) and the European Cosmetics Directory. Products include blends for relaxation, stress relief, stretch marks, perineal care, preparation for birth and skincare oils for babies (no essential oils).

Your greatest achievements? Over the last eight years we have launched two websites and have been approved to sell our products on Amazon and Not on the High Street. We have set up distribution in Thailand and have a Swedish distributor to sell the products across Scandinavia. After gaining the help of a business mentor, we have also eventually managed to get our pricing structure right, helping to grow the business much more successfully.

Your biggest mistake? Not selling on the correct advertising platforms.

How has your business evolved since you first started? We have increased our sales by changing to better advertising platforms, getting our products in front of our target market. We have kept up with the changes in social media and now use a variety of social media methods of advertising.

What is the best thing about working for yourself? Being in control of your working life.

What causes you most difficulty in running your own business? Never having enough time off. Learning how and what to prioritise, as there are so many aspects to running a business.

What advice would you give to a midwife/doula who is just setting out in the commercial world? Use the advice that is available from libraries and the various sources of government advice, especially when you are first starting up.

2

Getting Started

Setting up your private practice

So…you have decided to set up your own business…but where do you start? It is vital to research what you want to do and how you want to do it. Do not be tempted to rush ahead with enthusiasm as this may cause you either to make mistakes (which can be costly) or to find you have to 'unpick' something you initiated too early. I have mentored many midwives who become so excited about branching out on their own that they forge ahead with ideas that are only partly thought-through, often with disastrous consequences (and I have also done it myself).

I was once invited to visit two midwives who had enthusiastically set up a small centre offering antenatal classes and complementary therapies. The centre was in a beautiful setting on a business park surrounded by woods with plenty of free parking, but it was outside the town centre and the walk from the bus stop on the main road would have been difficult for many women in late pregnancy. They had invested a lot of time and money in setting up the business, including committing to a year-long lease on the property and having their cars covered with the company logo and contact details. Their ideas were good but the centre offered no potential for expansion as the main room would only accommodate about six to eight people and there was only one small room suitable for individual consultations. Further, they had developed a partnership (but not set it out formally) with a therapist with whom they then had a serious disagreement, eventually leading them to disband the business and go their separate ways.

Having decided that you really do want to set up your own practice and having looked honestly at your reasons for doing so, start by making some concrete plans. Decide on the services you wish to provide and consider how you would like to provide them. Take time to think about things, leaving it for a while and going back with fresh eyes once you have had time to consolidate your ideas. You may wish to refer back to the activities you completed in Chapter 1 to help you with this.

Defining your business activities

It is important to define your proposed services in detail before going ahead. Try to identify *exactly* what you wish to offer – if you do not know, then neither will your clients understand what you are offering. It is counter-productive to include too many different elements at the start of your new venture and you need to be flexible enough that other services can be added later. Activity 2.1 may help you with this.

When I set up Expectancy, I made the mistake of trying to be all things to all my potential customers. I wanted to offer clinical services to pregnant women, as well as professional courses. Not only did I want to provide education for midwives, but also for doulas, antenatal teachers and therapists. This meant that I was trying to spread my colleagues and myself (and my limited advertising budget) across at least four different markets. Indeed, my adverts were completely unclear because we had tried to have a 'one size fits all' leaflet – which just did not work. Everyone was confused – including the team. It was only later that I made the decision to focus solely on offering professional courses preparing the students to provide their own clinical services that it started to make sense. When I finally decided to concentrate entirely on marketing courses and business services for midwives, there was a consequent substantial growth in income. If I had taken the time and put in the effort at the start to explore specifically what I wanted to do, I may have achieved success more quickly and more productively.

Be clear about what you intend to provide, both in the short term and the longer term. You cannot start everything at once, and your business will develop as you grow and gain a reputation, sometimes even leading you in a completely different direction. I know of one midwife who set up her practice to offer massage, aromatherapy and reflexology to pregnant women but who then completed a course in neurolinguistic programming (NLP), a form of psychological talking therapy. Her interest had always been in reproductive mental health (she had previously worked in the NHS as a mental health midwife) and she found that offering NLP and focusing on antenatal and postnatal depression, birth 'after-thoughts' and other emotional issues gave her a unique selling point (USP) which helped her business to grow in a different – and very successful – direction from her initial intentions.

ACTIVITY 2.1: Deciding on your proposed services

– Make a list of the services you are considering offering in your practice. You may want to refer to Box 1.1 in Chapter 1 to help you with this activity, or you may have some wonderfully unique ideas of your own that you wish to explore.

— Identify your reasons for the services on your list.

— Discuss your thoughts and plans with your family and your colleagues and if possible, talk about your ideas with potential consumers of your services. Is there a market in your area for what you want to offer, and will women pay for it? Be aware of what is available to women via your local NHS services. If you have decided to offer postnatal care and lactation services, be sure that you know how much – or how little – of this is provided by the local maternity services. It would, for example, be difficult, both in business and professional terms, to offer a service for women who want to avoid induction of labour by accessing complementary therapies if your local maternity unit has already implemented a post-dates pregnancy clinic for 'natural induction'. Similarly, although there may, nationally, be a three- to four-week wait for treatment of babies with tongue-tie, leading you to think you could offer this privately, it would not be financially viable if the NHS frenulotomy service in your area was fortunate enough to have a very short waiting list.

— Research the competition and look at ways in which you may be able to offer something different or better. Which service providers in your area are successful or more successful than others? Do they have a particular focus on how they market (sell) their services? Are there other midwives or doulas in your area already offering what you are considering? (See also Chapter 5 on marketing.)

When I was setting up my company, one thing that stood in my favour was that I was providing a service that was not available anywhere else at the time. No organisation, either in higher education or the NHS, or in the commercial sector, provided professional and academic courses specifically on maternity complementary therapies. There were a few courses available for complementary therapy practitioners who wanted to specialise in maternity work, but these tended to focus on reproductive anatomy and physiology, and teaching a few different aspects of the therapy that applied to pregnancy. Expectancy offered – and still does – a unique range of accredited courses that have never been offered elsewhere, although some minor competition is creeping in more recently. This factor gave Expectancy its USP.

It is important to identify the passions that drive you and how these relate to your values as you set up your business. Your personal professional philosophy will impact on the structure of your business, the ways in which you choose to work and the motivation to succeed in your practice. My personal professional philosophy of 'safety, professional accountability and evidence-based practice' is something on which I have built my academic and clinical reputation over my entire working life. I still adhere to this philosophy so tenaciously that, on occasions, it has meant less income and some lost opportunities for more business. A few years ago I was invited to teach in Beijing but, although the company wanted me to return, I declined because they were so commercially driven that their attitude to safety was completely at odds with my own. On the other hand, I have delivered courses for many NHS trusts and maternity units overseas that have consciously chosen my services precisely because of my emphasis on safety and accountability. Having a USP enables you to focus your marketing and to sell your services direct to potential clients who have made a deliberate decision to access what *you* have to offer rather than going elsewhere for similar services. Activities 2.2, 2.3 and 2.4 will help you define you USP for your personal philosophy and your goals.

♀ ACTIVITY 2.2: Defining your unique selling point (USP)

To define your USP, think through your proposed plans. Try to put yourself into the women's shoes and think about the services for which they may be searching, and their reasons for doing so:

- What do you *think* women want? Is this *actually* what they want?

Now think about the women who are your target clients:

- Are you aiming to provide services for all pregnant women and their families or for specific groups of this wide market?

- What problems are you attempting to solve by the services you offer? Are you considering specific skills or packages that women will want to access?

- What are the most significant benefits to your clients of engaging *you* to provide these services?

⚑ ACTIVITY 2.3: Defining your personal philosophy

— In your opinion, what values represent you?

— How would you define your personal and/or professional philosophy?

— To what extent do you feel that ethical guidelines are integral to your business?

— How do you feel your answers to the questions above will impact on your business?

✎ ACTIVITY 2.4: Defining your goals

Having decided what you wish to offer, this activity aims to help you work out what your short- and longer-term goals are for your business.

-   In relation to the potential services you identified in Activity 2.1, try now to differentiate them into those you wish to offer immediately and those that you might offer at a later stage. Your decisions may be based on a variety of factors, including whether you particularly enjoy providing this sort of service, local demand from women, cost of setting up (equipment, etc.) or a need for you to undertake further training.

-   Following on from Activity 2.2, what can you do to make your business unique? Do you have a USP and/or a personal professional philosophy?

-   How would you like your business and its contribution to society to be described by the outside world? Depending on your answer, this may have a bearing on the structure of your business – for example, you may decide to set up as a social enterprise rather than a limited company (see below, 'The structure of your business').

— What is your desired position in the market, and how do you intend to get there? Do you only want to work locally, or do you have grandiose ideas of becoming global?

— What ethical dilemmas do you anticipate in achieving your goals and vision?

The structure of your business

One of the key decisions in setting up a new business is its legal structure, which must be addressed at the outset. There are several ways of trading in business, each with different advantages and disadvantages. For most midwives and doulas starting out, this will come down to a decision between being a sole trader, establishing a partnership or registering as a limited company. Other structures that may fit with your business objectives include social enterprises, charitable organisations, franchising and licensing.

Sole trader

This is a simple system in which you charge for your services, are paid direct by your clients (income) and account for your costs (outgoings). You can set up simply and start trading immediately, subject only to being in possession of the requisite skills, knowledge, insurance and maternity- or therapy-specific requirements. There is little administration to do and you are totally in control of how, when and where you work. You can adapt your services and the way you work as you go along without the need for lengthy bureaucratic processes that are inherent in a large organisation. (For an example of a midwife operating as a sole trader, see 'Case study: Dianne Garland', page 92.)

From a legal perspective, being a sole trader means that you are self-employed. It is advisable to discuss with your accountant whether being a sole trader is the most cost-efficient way of running your business. If you are very successful, it is probably better to register as a limited company as this can have tax benefits and you also reap the benefits of limited liability in the event of any debts (see below); it is, however, possible to move from being a sole trader to becoming a limited company at a later date. As a sole trader, you are personally liable for any and all losses your business may make and, if these are substantial, it could mean using some of your personal savings to pay creditors to whom you owe money. For example, you may decide to hire a specialist therapy chair or couch, but if you are unable to pay the rental fees and your business fails, you would be bound to pay the outstanding balance for the duration of the terms of the agreement. In the worst-case scenario, this could mean that your home, personal savings and other assets are under threat as these could be used to pay for major debts you have incurred. It can also be difficult to obtain a loan or a mortgage, as most lenders require you to present them with at least three years' accounts demonstrating that your personal income is sufficient to cover the loan and that you are not a credit risk. This can make future growth more difficult. You will also be less able to take advantage of economies of scale, for example, buying in bulk, because your cash flow is likely to be much tighter. This can mean that you have to charge more for your services than others offering similar services within a larger organisation, such as an established clinic set-up.

On a personal level, your time is not infinite, and the scope and growth of your business will be limited by only having the same number of hours as those with which you started. This is one of the main barriers to growth amongst sole traders who provide a service rather than those who sell products. On the plus side, many of your clients will enjoy the personal touch that comes with dealing solely with one person. Your clientele will choose you because of who you are, as much as for what you offer. This will help your reputation to grow and clients will come from word-of-mouth referrals, one of the best forms of advertising.

Whilst sole trader arrangements may suit many midwives and doulas when they first set up in business, it can be lonely working on your own and you may miss the camaraderie of being with colleagues on a day-to-day basis. It is easy to become out-of-date with important issues related to maternity care and working with pregnant and childbearing women. In many respects, a sole trader arrangement may seem to be the easy option, but it is wise to define your long-term goals right from the start. If you have plans, however tentative, to grow your business, perhaps eventually intending to open your own clinic, it is better to start now with one of the more formal business structures. Yes, it can be daunting and time-consuming, and you may be overwhelmed with bureaucratic processes, but it may be better to do it now than to get halfway through and then find that you have to change everything. Making your business a formal legal entity will also instil in you a sense of total commitment to the venture – the more difficult or expensive it is, the more effort you will put in to making it a success. If you start with a small business offering just occasional consultations fitted around your current work, the need to bring in an income may be more easily achieved by staying with or returning to your previous employment.

Partnership

In this system, you and one or more colleagues set up a business as partners. This means that costs, working times, holiday and sickness cover, administration and losses are shared equally. Partners often complement each other and the business may thrive because you can offer a variety of related services and there is professional and business interaction and the sharing of ideas.

The partners all contribute to the business start-up capital (finance), so the more partners there are, the more money can be put into the business, facilitating greater flexibility and potential for growth. This, in turn, helps to achieve greater profit, which is then shared equally between the partners. The business is generally easy to set up, manage and run, and partnerships are less strictly regulated by government than limited companies. The partners share responsibility for the running of the business, whilst generally complementing each other in terms of skills and approach.

However, a solicitor should be involved in helping you to set up the business, and a written contract is *absolutely essential*, particularly as the circumstances of one person may change or you may experience conflicts of ideas. This is especially important if your intended colleague is also a friend or family member. However close you are now, being in business together can change that and – unfortunately – you must be prepared for every eventuality. The deed of partnership should include not only the financial elements of the business, but also the processes to be followed in the event that one or more of the partners wishes to withdraw, for any reason, or if the business needs to be dissolved. Disagreements happen in all organisations but may have more disastrous personal consequences if the business has not been legally delineated. It is possible that each partner has different ideas on how the business should be run, the responsibilities of each person involved and the overall vision for the business.

As with sole traders, each partner is required to register as being self-employed and to pay personal tax to Her Majesty's Revenue & Customs (HMRC) via the annual self-assessment return. This can be a barrier to business growth because the more income the partnership makes, the more tax liability each partner will have. In the event of a very successful business, it is usually more tax efficient to set up as a limited company (see below).

With an ordinary partnership, each partner shares the liability and financial risks of the business. An option is to form a limited liability partnership in which each partner has the protection of only being responsible for her/his share of any losses, and not for any financial shortcomings of the partners. This is similar to a limited company, but provides a little more flexibility.

Limited company

A limited company is a business in which the liability for losses is limited to the company itself and shareholders are not personally liable: large assets such as houses, pensions and other savings remain the property of the individual. There are two types of limited company – public (PLC) and private. Public limited companies have at least two shareholders and at least £50,000 worth of shares issued, and are generally floated on the stock market; they include large national companies such as British Petroleum and Virgin Media PLC, for example.

It is sometimes erroneously believed that a limited company is only for larger start-ups such as establishing your own clinic or purchasing an existing large business. However, if your plans include substantial growth in a relatively short period of time, registering as a limited company should be considered at the outset, even though it may seem daunting. When I was first looking for an accountant, I was advised to register Expectancy as a limited company without really understanding the implications. For the first few years of my business I thought it had been a poor move because it just seemed to bring more paperwork and the scary threat of being fined huge amounts of money if accounts were submitted late to HMRC. However, I would advise you to consider becoming a limited company if you have big plans, not least because it ensures your commitment to the venture more substantially than being a sole trader.

A limited company is seen as a legal entity in its own right and can be subject to legal action in the same way as an individual. It survives in law after the withdrawal or death of the shareholders. A solicitor and an accountant are required to help you set up a limited company. It is by far the safest way of setting up a business, but incurs the heaviest workload in terms of administration. For your personal tax affairs, you are actually employed by the limited company and do not come into the same category as self-employed people running their own businesses (sole traders).

Under the Companies Act 2006, a limited company must be registered with Companies House and have at least one director (you) who runs the business. There also needs to be a company secretary, responsible for ensuring that the company complies with legal and financial governance, although this can be the same person as one of the directors. The directors and any other people involved in the company own shares (shareholders) and reap the benefits of any profits, usually paid in the form of dividends over the following year.

The company is taxed on any profits (Corporation Tax of 20% at the time of writing), but this can often be advantageous over being a sole trader in which you would be taxed on your whole income. An annual return must be filed to both Companies House and HMRC. There are other tax advantages of being a limited company, for example, being able to claim for use of part of your home as an office or clinic room, although it is not generally tax efficient to run a company car. Becoming a limited company means that the shareholders establish and manage the business as they wish, retaining control and flexibility over the day-to-day running.

Social enterprise

The aim of a social enterprise is usually one of philanthropy, that is, to give something of value to the local, national or international community. For those who have worked within the NHS system, in which healthcare is free at the point of access for patients and clients, this model can help you to overcome the issue of charging for your services whilst enabling you to care for women in a way that fits with your personal philosophy and without the constraints of a cumbersome organisation. Social enterprises are likely to be more acceptable and better supported by midwives and other staff working in the conventional maternity services, because the care given to women is usually free of charge or heavily subsidised. Although social enterprises will generate income, they do not tend to become wealthy, since the profit is usually ploughed back into the business for the benefit of its consumers.

Working in a social enterprise provides opportunities for flexibility and the provision of individualised care, and the services may be more cost-effective than similar services offered by a commercial organisation. It is often easier to obtain funding to establish a social enterprise, and there are many incentives and benefits from the government that support them. Marketing can also be easier as media will welcome an organisation that sets out to tackle a social issue by offering an innovative solution. Conversely, the need to compete within the commercial sector can sometimes lead to economic failure of the enterprise, particularly as it can be difficult to balance the financial and social aims of the organisation.[1]

An example of a social enterprise in midwifery is One to One Midwives,[2] which contracts with NHS trusts to provide maternity services to specified groups of women in different areas. One to One is based mainly in the North East of England but also has a team in Essex. It was established by Jo Parkington, both for the benefit of women and to enable midwives to work autonomously and in partnership with parents. She had initially started the business as a limited company but later changed to a social enterprise, with indemnity insurance cover provided by the NHS Litigation Authority. The NHS pays One to One Midwives and the services are free to the women, facilitating the provision of individualised maternity care to women from all social strata, not just that proportion of the community that can afford to pay for it. This is distinctly different from independent midwifery, although the way in which the midwives work is similar to the model adopted by self-employed midwives.

Another organisation set up as a social enterprise is Neighbourhood Midwives[3] in London and the South East of England. It is an employee-owned mutual organisation in which all the midwives contribute to the way in which the company works. Private services are available to women wishing to pay but free-at-the-point-of-access care is also provided for women in the Waltham Forest area of East London, for which the local NHS trust pays. This is a pilot scheme and the aim is to spread the system out across other areas of the country.

Charitable organisation

Some businesses with a social conscience set up as charitable foundations, but it is essential to do this for the right reasons and not simply to promote your business. There is a huge amount of paperwork

---

1   For government information on setting up a social enterprise, see www.gov.uk/set-up-a-social-enterprise
2   www.onetoonemidwives.org
3   www.neighbourhoodmidwives.org.uk/news/neighbourhood-midwives-a-brief-history

to be completed before and after setting up as a charity. The charity must exist only for the public benefit and any income above a certain level must be filed for public inspection with the Charity Commission (England and Wales) or the Office of the Scottish Charity Regulator in Scotland. It is vital to plan any funding requests as monies given to the charity cannot be returned. Appointed trustees must act only in the best interests of the charity and do not have nearly as much control over the business of the charity as other business structures. There are specific tax rules for charitable organisations and a charity should not be considered a tax-free zone. There are also regulations around Gift Aid, direct tax and Value Added Tax (VAT), which must be considered before transferring funds or making important strategic decisions. Although setting up a charitable foundation may resonate with your personal and professional philosophies, it is not generally considered a way of making money for yourself. If you have a particularly strong social conscience, it may be wiser to consider setting up as a social enterprise.

Franchise

A franchise is a system in which an established business offers the opportunity to individuals to run their own business but under the business name of the franchisor (owner). Many high street businesses are run as franchises, including McDonald's and other fast food outlets, petrol stations and parcel delivery operators. The advantage to the franchisee (the person who buys a franchise) is that they have the right to use the trade name and trademark of the parent company as well as certain business processes, under the supervision and with the support of the franchisor whilst essentially owning their own business.

Buying a franchise can be a good way of getting into business ownership because the franchisor usually provides all the necessary training – after all, it is in their best interests to make sure the franchisee is successful. It is also often much less expensive to set up a franchise than to start a business from scratch, and the reputation of the franchise name usually results in a good income. On the other hand, it can be costly: buying into a global franchise such as McDonald's, which may bring in a multi-million dollar income, requires assets of around three-quarters of a million dollars at the outset, although other franchises may be available for as little as £5000. The disadvantage is that there is much less flexibility and the franchisee is not encouraged to be creative with the business, since all franchise outlets must offer the same products or services. Any profit you make must be shared with the franchisor, and you may be constrained by requirements to use particular suppliers, where you operate and how you are permitted to expand. Furthermore, the franchisor does not have to renew the agreement at the end of the term, but there are often legal restrictions on setting up similar services by yourself after the end of the term of the agreement. I know of one business colleague who bought into a virtual assistant franchise who became very disillusioned by the practices within the parent company. Unfortunately, when she tried to extricate herself from the agreement, she found that she was bound by the terms of the agreement and that she could not act as an independent virtual assistant for another two years.

If the franchise option appeals to you, be sure to clarify whether the business is a member of the British Franchise Association (BFA).[4] Examples of existing maternity-related franchise operations include several maternity clothing companies and nanny agencies, and the Daisy Foundation for its Lazy Daisy antenatal classes.[5]

On the other hand, you may have ideas to franchise your own business once it grows. To do this you must have a proven track record and a successful business with a product or service that is identifiable and marketable. There are complicated procedures to be undertaken in order to set up a franchise, and you must meet specified criteria to register with the BFA. You will need to look carefully at your business model and demonstrate to potential franchisees that they will be able to build a successful and financially rewarding business from it. It is normal practice to run a pilot scheme for at least a year after making the decision to franchise. Franchising is a good way to grow your business in the long run, but you must be prepared to monitor your franchisees to ensure that they adhere to your principles and practices.

---

4   www.thebfa.org
5   www.femalefranchise.co.uk/CaseStudies/LazyDaisy/1826

Licensed practitioner

Becoming a licensed practitioner is similar to a franchise but a simpler model. It taps into the ideas already established by someone with a reputation in the field, but allows you more flexibility than with a franchise to develop the business as your own. You also benefit from the support and mentoring of the parent company, both in business matters and the services or products offered. It is usually considerably cheaper than either setting up your own business or buying into a franchise (typically around £1000–£5000, depending on the type of business), but allows licensees to benefit from the business name of the licensor. The terms of agreement are usually shorter and less restrictive than for a franchise. Several caring professions work on preparing students to become licensed practitioners for the organisation, including life coaches, NLP practitioners and other therapists.

My own company, Expectancy,[6] offers a Licensed Consultancy scheme for midwives who have completed a programme of education (Diploma in Midwifery Complementary Therapies or Certificate in Midwifery Acupuncture) together with comprehensive business training. This enables the midwife to have ongoing support to set up, establish and maintain their own practice, to join a growing network of like-minded midwives in business, and to receive mentoring and advice on clinical issues that they may encounter in private practice.

Case study: Cassie Marnoch RM Dip HE Midwifery

Nueva Vida Therapies (www.facebook.com/nuevavidatherapies) is based in South East England, in the Sevenoaks and Tunbridge Wells area.

I started my business in November 2016. I'd already left full-time employment as a midwife in the NHS due to long-term sickness and wanted to continue working with women and their families, but on my own terms. I knew that once I'd left the NHS I'd never be going back, and still wanted to be a midwife. Working this way allows me to give the time and care I'm passionate about for women and families. I completed several courses to help me prepare, including a Diploma in Midwifery Complementary Therapies, a Certificate in Midwifery Acupuncture and more recently, neurolinguistic programming (NLP).

6   http://expectancy.co.uk/business

I provide a range of pregnancy services including aromatherapy, reflex zone therapy (a clinical style of reflexology) and massage for pregnancy issues such as nausea and vomiting or backache, as well as for relaxation. I offer sessions to teach women with breech presentation how to perform moxibustion safely and acupuncture for a whole variety of antenatal and postnatal situations. I also provide preparation for labour for individuals and in group sessions and enhanced antenatal care packages. I have a particular interest in mental health issues and post-traumatic stress disorder (PTSD), both in parents and healthcare professionals, and use NLP to help with these problems. I visit women in their own homes and also hire a room in a centre two days a week. Although I'm currently still earning less than £20,000, things are definitely on the up, and the next year looks to be very successful.

Your greatest achievements? In all honesty, it's actually being a year down the line and still having a business! It's not where I want it to be yet but I have a great base to work from and make it amazing. I hardly spent anything in setting up the business (except for training courses and a small amount on marketing – leaflets, website, networking, etc.).

Your biggest mistake? Not being consistent with driving it forward. Some of that has been due to health reasons, but even so, I wish I'd been more consistent.

How has your business evolved since you first started? I've rebranded and have a more definite focus on the areas I want to specialise in. From what I thought it would be at the beginning to where it's heading now is completely different!

What is the best thing about working for yourself? Time. Time to actually listen to and be with women. Sometimes I do nothing more than allow them to offload in a quiet and supported environment, and the difference that small thing makes is amazing. No more 'conveyor belt' midwifery for me or for those I work with.

What causes you most difficulty in running your own business? The change from having a wage at the end of every month to having to actually put a value on yourself is a difficult transition, and keeping abreast of changes in areas such as data protection is definitely challenging!

What advice would you give to a midwife/doula who is just setting out in the commercial world? Go for it! Be prepared to be fluid in your approach – if one thing doesn't work, then try something else until you find what does for you and the area you work in. *Network*, the most important thing I've done. I really didn't think it was for me and was dragged to my first meeting kicking and screaming, but I'm so glad I was! I've met some amazing people along the way, some to collaborate with, some to be friends with and others to buy from. It doesn't have to be another expense; there are some great networking groups that cost you the price of a coffee whilst you're there. Social media is great, but face-to-face is really important for people to really connect with you. Value yourself and remember it's not just the treatment/care that people are buying. It's also you, your experience, education, skills and time.

Modes of delivering your private practice

There are several ways in which you can establish yourself as an independent practitioner offering maternity-related services, each with various advantages and disadvantages. This will be affected partly by the legal structure you have chosen and whether you are working alone or in conjunction with others, as well as the geographical and social demographics of your chosen area of work. You may wish to practise from your own home, work peripatetically or from a hired clinic room, or you may have plans to open your own premises.

Working from home

This is one of the easiest and cheapest ways of starting your business. If you choose to run your private practice from home, you have flexibility in deciding when and how you work and you have complete control over your working area. There is no need to travel to a place of work or to clients' homes to provide treatments, saving on the costs, time and stress of travel, with the unpredictability of excessive traffic. This means that you may be able to see more women in a day. Conversely, you may be distracted by family noise and movement around the house, such as the telephone ringing or the dog barking. In turn, your work life may encroach into your home, with equipment spilling over into rooms other than the one you use for treatments. You will need to be firm with clients about which door they use for access, and you will need to keep your home tidy and professional looking, including access to a toilet. For example, if a client needs to enter your treatment room through your hallway, keep it free of clutter. Ideally, you should have a dedicated room, separated from the main living areas, preferably on the ground floor, and with access to a toilet that is not part of the main family bathroom.

I have a business colleague who works as a Bowen Technique therapist and has set up a clinic room in a beautiful wooden hut in the garden. The room is lovely, with restful décor and plenty of space. However, she lives in a very small terraced house, and in order to reach the clinic room, you have to go through her galley kitchen, which is often extremely untidy and smells of cooking. The only access to a toilet for clients is to use the tiny downstairs bathroom in the house, which is the only one available and therefore used by the whole family. Unfortunately, this does not give a good first impression to clients and may be off-putting to some. I also know of a midwife in Wales who has spent several thousand pounds on converting her garage to a beautiful treatment room, with hot and cold running water and a toilet. Access is via a dedicated door that does not intrude on the family and the whole area is clean, clinical, yet homely and extremely professional.

Some people find it liberating, less stressful and more productive to work from home, but it can also be very lonely if you prefer the social interaction of being with colleagues. You could potentially not leave the house on some days, even though you are seeing clients and meeting people. It is important to ensure that you get out each day for some fresh air and exercise; otherwise you might find that you become too sedentary. It is essential to overcome the lack of daily exposure to colleagues by networking with both the midwifery and/or doula communities and amongst local business colleagues. You may also be more at risk of theft or even assault if you are alone in the house, and may decide only to work when someone else is nearby. You do, however, have the flexibility and opportunity to take a break from the workplace for a short time.

You need to be disciplined when working from home, both in achieving what you need to do and in 'switching off'. For many it can be difficult to stop thinking about what you need to do, since your work and home life are physically in the same building. Try to identify when and how you work best, set yourself a working day and close the door on your work environment once you reach the cut-off time. This is not easy; however, it is not only important for you to separate your work and home life, but also to give the message to clients that you may not always be immediately available to them. Make a pledge not to answer the telephone or emails out of hours, in the same way you would if off-duty from your job in the NHS or a large company. Similarly, when you are officially working, try to avoid getting involved in household chores such as putting the washing machine on or vacuuming the carpets (it can be difficult!). Working from home enables you to take time out of the working day to fetch children from school or go to the gym, but this should be *allocated* time, not just done *ad hoc* because you are bored with the task in hand. It can also feel as if work never ends and there may be a temptation for you to work long hours, completing your records, audits or ordering of new stock once you have finished seeing your clients for the day. Remember, if you were employed there would be a finite point at which your working day finished – and one of the reasons that could have influenced your decision to set up your own practice may have been the incessant workload and never finishing on time.

You will need to inform your mortgage provider and change your household insurance cover to account for use of part of it as a business, and it would be advisable to obtain public liability insurance in case someone has an accident on your premises. The use of a dedicated room at home can be offset against tax, taking into account a proportion of your gas and electricity usage, mortgage, telephone and broadband costs, but this may not be the case if you use the treatment room for other purposes. From a professional point of view, the room should, in any case, be kept clean and fresh, without allowing your children, the cat or cooking odours to be admitted. You may also be liable for business rates for the proportion of the house used for your business.

Mobile practice

Many therapists and other professionals providing services to individuals choose to work peripatetically, visiting clients in their homes rather than inviting them to their own (although some provide both options). Essentially running costs are low and the costs of travel can (and should) be incorporated into the costs of treatments (see Chapter 4 on setting prices). Your work and home life are separate, both physically and, to a certain extent, mentally, although some of your administrative work will need to be done at home. The time that you spend on driving to your first destination, travelling between visits and returning home from your last location should all be factored into your costs *and* the duration of your working day. Further, driving between the locations of different clients can be time-consuming and adversely affected by heavy traffic, and you will be able to see less clients in a day than if they came to you. This can be stressful and you may not be at your best as you become increasingly tired throughout the day. You may also need to plan your visits according to the geographical location of each client. It is not time- or cost-efficient to drive across town for one client only to have to drive back again for the next. And as with community midwifery, it may be difficult to ask to use the lavatory in some houses, or you may not find suitable places to eat lunch except in the car.

Your car must be kept in good working order to avoid unanticipated breakdowns, and you will need to change your car insurance to business use, although this may not always cost more than insurance for commuting and social use. However, if you do not change your insurance and are in an accident, you can be prosecuted if it is found that you were engaged in work-related activities.

Take into account your personal security and leave a 'whereabouts' list with someone at home in case your return is delayed. It is useful to invest in an up-to-date satellite navigation system for your car (a legitimate business expense), or use an online one via your mobile telephone. Getting lost trying to find your destination will only add to your stress. Indeed, you should always have your mobile telephone with you and keep a spare charger cable in the car for use in an emergency.

Although many women like the idea of visits at home, you have no control over the environment into which you are going. There may be toddlers running around or the television may be on. This can be distracting for you and is not the best environment for the woman if the purpose of your visit is to provide relaxation treatments or information and counselling-type consultations. You may also have large amounts of equipment to transport into clients' homes, which can be tedious and risks causing you injury if heavy; some equipment may be quite cumbersome and you may have to consider how you stack everything in your vehicle to prioritise accessibility.

Renting rooms in a clinic

This is a relatively low-cost option and all the legal issues are normally covered by the practice. For example, a well-established clinic should have public liability insurance cover in place – and you should check this when enquiring about room availability. You will have opportunities for referrals and there are usually a receptionist and other services available. On the other hand, you have no control over the tenancy or rental costs or even the room décor or layout. You will usually have to pay for room rental even when you have no clients – and this may include your holidays and any time that you are unwell. Further, you have no control over the reputation of the clinic – any negative aspects may be seen to relate to all practitioners associated with the clinic. In addition, be careful to choose somewhere that fits with your personal philosophy and the way that you want to work. For example, if you are providing clinical treatments or midwifery services, you may not wish to work from a centre that is essentially offering beauty therapy or hairdressing. I know of a homeopath who rented rooms in a hairdressing salon that also offered some beauty therapy, but her time there was short-lived because the smells of the various chemicals used for hair treatments was so overpowering and she was concerned that they may affect the homeopathic remedies she was prescribing for her clients (a distinct possibility since homeopathic medicines are chemically very fragile and can be inactivated by strong odours). It may be wise to search for rooms in a general practitioner's (GP) surgery, chiropractic clinic or large complementary medicine clinic that offers a range of practitioners of credible therapies. This will also give you some valuable networking opportunities and the possibility of cross-referrals.

Find out how you will be charged for the room: most clinics charge by the hour or session, such as an afternoon of perhaps three hours' duration. Some may charge a percentage of your income whilst in the clinic – which is not particularly fair if your fees reflect a variety of different services. A friend with her own complementary therapy business wanted to rent a room from a colleague who ran a clinic so that she could offer clinical reflexology and massage for cancer patients. The room rental was charged at 33 per cent of the takings. However, because she was offering specialist treatments for lymphoedema and other cancer-related complications, the fees were considerably more than standard relaxation treatments offered by other practitioners using the clinic. Thus, her fees for the room were more than her colleagues', despite the fact that all those renting a room were provided with exactly the same facilities. On the days my friend used the clinic, the owner was absent so she had to open up, answer the door and close the clinic herself. She also found the rooms were so disorganised when she arrived that she needed to clean and tidy everywhere before she could start each clinic session. Needless to say, she did not stay there long!

Similarly, check the lease contract: it may be wise to ask a solicitor to check it for you before you sign it, especially if it appears complicated. Many clinics will require you to commit to a length of time, perhaps six months or a year, and to give notice if you wish to leave; this may be one month's notice or longer. Clarify precisely what will be provided for you – and what will not be provided. This relates to equipment available in the room, facilities for your clients whilst waiting to see you, personnel such as receptionist availability and whether your room will be cleaned or you are expected to clean it yourself.

Buying an existing practice

If you choose to purchase someone else's business, it is basically ready-made for you. Buying an existing practice gives you an instant supply of clients, with credibility if the previous owner was good (although you usually pay for this financially in the form of 'goodwill' in addition to the purchase price of the business). Conversely, it is essential to question the owner's reasons for selling the business at this time: there may be genuine personal or business reasons, but if the business has failed, consider issues such as the location and the local population's demand for services that you wish to offer. Also find out if any existing staff contracts may impact on your business, or if there is a sitting tenant in the flat above. Also bear in mind that you may initially lose clients if your style, personality, prices or selection of treatments are different from the previous owner's, and it can take time to build up your own clientele.

One advantage is that the clinic is likely to be already set up for clinical work, with individual treatment rooms, disabled access, kitchen and toilet facilities, a waiting area and staff area. Alternatively, you may wish to, or need to, change the structural layout of the building (with local authority planning permission) and the décor. You may also need to apply to the local council for a change of use, depending on the services offered there by the previous owner and the nature of your own intended services. Business premises are classified by local councils according to their usage, grouped from class A (shops, financial services, food and drink), B (business services and industrial), C (hotels and residential institutions) to class D, which is divided into D1 and D2, the latter relating to assembly and leisure services.

Properties that provide non-residential services including medical or health services, nurseries or crèches, educational institutions, libraries, museums and places of worship are classified as class D1. One independent midwife colleague of mine, who wanted to establish a designated centre for midwifery consultations, antenatal classes and complementary therapies, found a baby equipment shop in a local high street that seemed to be an ideal location.[7] Unfortunately, the local council declined to change the usage from a shop (A1) to a clinic (D1) because they were committed to a high street with a good selection of shops. However, they agreed that she could provide her desired services in the building on condition that the shop front remained.

---

7   www.bababoom-boutique.co.uk

She therefore decided to sell baby equipment, maternity clothing and other products suitable for expectant mothers, which attracted women into the shop and actually helped to grow her other services.

Establishing your own clinic

If you choose to establish a totally new venture you will have total autonomy and security and will be able to develop a considerable asset for sale if you eventually decide to withdraw from the business. Rooms can be hired out to other practitioners, bringing in additional income. However, it is very expensive to set up from scratch. You may need planning permission for change of use to D1, and you are required to comply with all health and safety legislation, which may require structural changes to the building, for example, the provision of disabled access if not already available. Many of the principles discussed above, in the section on buying an existing business, apply to setting up your own clinic.

Contracting with the NHS

You could consider approaching an NHS trust to offer your services on their premises as a fee-paying service for the women booked for delivery in that unit. Alternatively you could negotiate a contract with the NHS unit (or a private maternity unit) for the NHS to pay you to provide a service that is free to the women. These options mean that you are in a familiar setting, appropriate for your needs – for example, you may be able to use the antenatal clinic in the evenings, which is ideal for seeing your clients. However, you have to be very clear which 'hat' you are wearing, most especially if you do this in the unit where you are still working as a midwife (or if you have been working there but have now resigned). It is best to try to offer a service that is not currently available in the NHS, for example, post-dates pregnancy natural induction or specialist antenatal 'massage for birth' classes (see also Chapter 3 on conflicts of interest).

The Any Qualified Provider (AQP) scheme is a means of commissioning certain NHS services in England. Clinical Commissioning Groups (CCGs) determine the services to be commissioned as AQP; the intention is to increase patient choice. All providers must meet the qualification criteria set for a particular service. You need to develop a comprehensive proposal under the AQP system and submit this. It can take quite some time to receive feedback, be invited for a meeting or be given a definitive 'accept' or 'reject' answer. In maternity care, antenatal education and breastfeeding support services have been available under the AQP system since 2014, but the time may now be right for other maternity-related services to be offered to individual CCGs under this system, particularly given the advent of the Personal Maternity Care Budget (PMCB) scheme.

✎ ACTIVITY 2.3: Deciding on the structure of your business and how you wish to work

- What are your initial thoughts on how you would prefer to structure your business? Do you wish to be a sole trader, engage in a partnership, become a limited company or strive for a social enterprise or other format? Try to identify your reasons for your initial decision.

- Make a list of the pros and cons of your proposed structure.

- Now refer back to your plans outlined in Activities 1.1 and 1.2 and consider your longer-term goals. What effect could your proposed business structure potentially have on your long-term plans? Think again about the business structure and consider whether you might be wise to change this to a different structure.

- How would you like to work in the first two years of your business? Do you want to work from home or peripatetically? Do you have plans to open your own centre? Identify your reasons for your choice.

- Again, referring to your long-term plans, will you need to make changes after a couple of years if you decide on working one way and then need to change later to fit in with your goals?

Choosing a name for your business

Having a business name gives your practice an identity that enables potential clients to find you. Choosing a name can be exciting and fun but again, look at your long-term plans before deciding definitively. You do not want to start with a restrictive name that implies the services you offer at the outset, only to find later that you need to change the name to reflect better the newer services you have introduced. One midwife whose passion was aromatherapy chose a name with the word 'aroma' in it, but found, within a very short period of time, that she was being asked for other services such as moxibustion for breech presentation. Although she chose not to change the name, she then had to look carefully at how she marketed her services in order to tell women that she offered more than just aromatherapy in pregnancy.

Conversely, you do not want to select a business name that is so broad that potential clients do not understand what you offer. Do not try to be clever or funny with words – be clear and avoid professional terminology (this also applies to marketing). *You* may know what you mean by words such as 'complementary therapies', but will the women needing your services understand the term? In this example, they will be searching online for terms such as 'aromatherapy in pregnancy'.

Similarly, using your own name, which is a popular option for many non-pregnancy-related businesses, does not necessarily tell your customers what you do unless you also add a word related to the services you intend to offer (e.g., John Smith Builders). Even if you are well known within your professional field (midwifery or doula work), the women searching for your services are unlikely to have heard of you; they will not search for your name but rather for the service they require. Of course, you *are* the identity of your business, but it can take some time to build up your reputation.

The name of your business needs to be short, precise and memorable. Although I was very well known in the midwifery and complementary therapy professional areas when I started my company, I actively chose not to use my name as the company name. I had had the idea for the name for some time and it was intended to be an acronym for **EX**pectant **P**arents' **C**omplementary **T**herapies consult**ANCY** – but that was too wordy. It does, however, condense nicely to 'Expectancy' – which easily implies that it is something to do with pregnancy (although searching for the term 'expectancy' on the internet initially seemed to focus on 'life expectancy').

You might want to think about where your business will be placed in any advertising you may do. It is not uncommon to see taxi firms called 'Abba taxis' or similar because this places them, alphabetically, at the beginning of any list of taxi firms. If you use a word starting with 'w' you will be near the end of a list, although perhaps something beginning with 'z' stands out even though it places you at the very end of an alphabetical list.

Your business name should be easy to pronounce and spell. An example that is frequently seen in advertisements, even on shop fronts and banners, is the use of the words 'complementary therapies', with the first word spelled as 'complimentary'. This is not only grammatically incorrect but also unprofessional, and the confusion over the correct spelling may mean that prospective clients searching online may not find you as easily as someone else offering maternity complementary therapies. The use of hyphens or unnecessary punctuation marks can also confuse people when searching online or on social media.

If you intend to register as a limited company with Companies House (see below), there are some legal constraints on the choice of your business name – and you are not permitted to add the word 'limited' to your business name unless you *have* registered as a limited company. You must be very careful about use of the words 'midwife' or 'midwifery', which are legally protected titles; you will need to obtain from the Nursing and Midwifery Council (NMC) a *Certificate of No Objection* to use these words in your business name (or 'health visitor', 'health visiting', 'nurse' or 'nursing' and other statutorily regulated professional terms). In addition you may not use words such as 'British', 'UK' or any word that implies an association with a government or official agency within the four countries of the United Kingdom. Similarly, you must avoid words such as 'association', 'council', 'charitable', 'federation', 'health centre', 'health service', 'institution' or 'society' without a Certificate of No Objection from the relevant authority.

You are not permitted to choose the same name as another business registered with Companies House.[8] This is not a legal requirement if you choose not to operate as a limited company, but it is wise to undertake a comprehensive online search for businesses that may have similar names or use similar words as those you are considering. Common words used in pregnancy-related businesses include 'natal' and 'mama'. This should be a search that not only applies to your local

8   https://beta.companieshouse.gov.uk/company-name-availability

area, but also nationally and even internationally, depending on the type of business and how far you intend to offer your services.

Some companies trademark their name to prevent others using it. You can search online to see if there is already a registered company using your proposed name.[9] It may not be essential to trademark your business name when you first start, but as you become more well known and established, you may choose to do so. I had been in business for six years before I trademarked 'Expectancy' and I chose to do so at this time because I was about to teach in China. In this case I applied for – and received – an international trademark to protect my intellectual property rights.

Before confirming the name, check whether your preferred domain name is available for your website and email address. This is another way of searching for private practice names that may be similar to the one you are considering. You can request a '.co.uk' or '.com' web address or a more geographically specific one such as '.wales' or '.scot'. When searching for your chosen domain name, it may be wise to purchase all similar domains such as .net, .org, etc. to prevent others from buying them. This could lead to confusion for users and possibly adversely affect your reputation or your business.

Choosing a locality for your practice

You are required to have a formal business address, even if you work from your home. If you opt for limited company status you must have a legally registered address, although this may not be a correspondence address. Many limited company directors (including me) use their accountant's address as the registered address, yet the business may be located many miles away. Take care if you are working from home – you may not wish to have your personal address on your website, and it is wise to refer only to your geographical area. Of course your clients will know where you live once they come for their first consultation, but you will have greater peace of mind about online security.

If you are providing consultations in women's own homes, you will need to include a geographical area within which you are prepared to travel, so this gives you more flexibility and informs your potential

9   www.gov.uk/search-for-trademark

clients of your location right from the start. You may choose to provide some consultations by Skype or a similar online platform, in which case your geographical location is less relevant.

If you are considering setting up from scratch and are looking for premises, ensure that the venue is accessible by public transport, and that there is adequate (preferably free or low-cost) parking. You will need a solicitor to deal with the legal aspects and possibly a chartered surveyor to confirm that the proposed property is safe and appropriate for your services. You may need to include the Care Quality Commission (CQC) in approving everything in your premises, from provision of emergency access to fire- and bacteria-repellent paint on the walls. An independent midwife friend who set up a birth centre had prolonged debates with the CQC because they required the centre to have a mortuary. This was because the birth centre was classified by the CQC as an acute hospital setting, even though my colleague was at pains to emphasise to the CQC that she really did not expect to have any deaths on her premises!

If you choose to establish a large enough practice that you can rent rooms to other practitioners, you must also clarify the legal relationship with those who lease space from you, and with your own staff. You must have in place guidelines and policies for the processes to follow in the event of disputes, complaints, professional conduct issues and health and safety issues, and will need additional insurance and organisational memberships to protect yourself, your business and those who enter it. If your business is expected to grow rapidly it may be wise to consider the services of a virtual receptionist or personal assistant who can field telephone calls, make appointments and manage your diary for you whilst leaving you time and space to go out and provide the clinical services.

Developing a business plan

It is essential to have a plan in mind for what you want to do with your business, even if it is not a formal written document. Developing and implementing strategic change is a skill that you will need for the duration of your business, and writing a business plan is the first step in this discipline. It is easy, once you start trading, to become engrossed in the day-to-day minutiae of running your practice, but you also need to look at the wider picture and the longer-term goals in order to achieve your vision. This is often referred to as 'working on' your business rather than 'working in' it – in other words, not simply doing the maternity-related work, but examining how you can take the business to the next step.

It will be necessary to write a business plan if you need to raise finance from the bank or another source of lending, or if you want to contract your services to the NHS or another organisation. However, even if you do not require external funding, developing a business plan is a valuable learning experience to help increase your understanding of the financial and practical aspects of starting your business. The process of writing your plan prior to setting up your business helps you to focus on what you want to achieve and how you are going to get there. You will need to have thought through the services you intend to offer and whether or not you believe the venture to be a viable option. This can only be achieved through researching the subject in depth, finding out what is available, what other people charge for similar services, what the local maternity unit offers and the demographics of your local area to determine if women will pay for your services.

It is important to format your document correctly and to be concise whilst providing sufficient information so that anyone else reading it can understand what you intend. Writing a business plan is similar to writing an academic essay, but you may need to adapt the way in which it is written and the language used, depending on its purpose. For example, is it for your own planning purposes only, for prospective clients or staff, to obtain funding, as an application to the council for premises or to an NHS maternity unit? Your passion must shine through and you need to be able to justify why you think your services are needed and why you care enough to provide them. A business plan should avoid maternity-related professional jargon so that it is easily understood by any sources of financial support you may approach, but also to focus on what your consumers (clients) want rather than on what you believe you are offering. Once you have written a full business plan you should also try to précis it to a single-sheet summary – both the full and condensed version may be necessary at different times. Boxes 2.4 and 2.5 summarise what needs to be included.

Once you have commenced trading you should review your business successes and possible failures annually, much in the same way as the annual review of practice that midwives undertake in the NHS. You can revisit your initial plan and revise it in line with the way your business is evolving.

There are many business websites available on the internet that provide advice on writing a business plan or proposal, and many also have free downloadable templates for you to adapt, although these are commonly intended solely for financial planning.[10] You may wish to pay for the services of someone who can write the plan for you, but do not be drawn into expensive contracts – do your own homework first and consider whether you can do this yourself and if possible, ask family and friends with their own businesses to advise you.

Box 2.4: A summary of the content of a business plan

Your business plan should include:

- *Vision:* What services will be offered and to which clients?
- *Mission:* Reasons for your business – philosophy and primary aims.
- *Objectives:* What results will you measure from the services you provide?
- *Strategy:* How will you build the business?
- *Action:* What do you need to do to fulfil your plan?

Box 2.5: Format of a full business plan to establish your business

- *Title page* with your business name, your name and relevance to the proposal (e.g., director), the date of the plan and your contact details (landline telephone, mobile telephone, email address, facsimile number, website address, postal or registered address, limited company number and VAT registration number, if appropriate).
- *Company logo* (not essential).

---

10 See www.gov.uk, which has links to many other business websites, and the Federation of Small Businesses' section on this at www.fsb.org.uk/resources/writing-a-business-plan

- *Contents page* with page numbers.

- *Executive summary:* This is essentially an introduction. It should be a brief overview of what you intend to offer and what you are attempting to achieve (similar to an abstract); it may be best to write this at the end as you may wish to summarise salient points from the rest of the document. It should be concise, logical and interesting and between 500 and 1000 words in length. The more detailed part of the business plan should reflect your executive summary and vice versa.

- *The structure of your business,* including the type of business, legal framework (sole trader, limited company), the number of people involved and their roles and responsibilities.

- *Background to the proposal:* This helps you to justify your ideas. Explain why you feel the service is needed and why women are likely to want to pay for it – in other words, this should be an analysis of the market that demonstrates the demand for your intended services. You should also identify some of the problems encountered by pregnant women and the negative effects these may have on them – for example, dissatisfaction with NHS care, the adverse physiological effects of stress in pregnancy, women's desire to expedite labour or a fear of being left alone in labour. Use references and statistics to support your discussion. This is the part that is most similar to writing an academic essay, but be concise and use appropriate language. For example, avoid professional terminology if you are seeking a financial loan, but write academically and professionally if you want to gain a contract with the NHS.

- *Identify what you intend to offer in your business:* Try to think in terms of what women want rather than what you feel they are demanding. For example, if you wish to offer treatments for women whose pregnancies are post-dates, the justification is that women wish to avoid medical induction of labour simply because they are 'overdue'. You do not need to describe the treatments or services you intend to offer – if necessary this can be included in a glossary or as an appendix. Identify the benefits that your proposal could offer to women, and anticipate any potential obstacles that may impact on your success. If you are approaching a maternity unit, show how contracting in your services could offer benefits for the unit such as cost savings, reduced intervention, etc.

- *Describe how you will set up your services,* including how, when, where and who will be involved. Be very clear about exactly how you intend to set up your services, with a time frame from the planning stage to implementation (start of trading). This section will help you to work out what is needed in terms of preparation, additional learning, and access to resources for things you are unable to do yourself, such as building a website.

- *Your sales and marketing strategy:* How will you tell people about your services and what costs are involved in this? Indeed, how do you know that women will want your services? In other words, justify how you will ensure sufficient business to earn enough money – and to be able to repay any lending if you wish to borrow finance. You also need to show that there is, in fact, a demand for your services and demonstrate where you see yourself in relation to the rest of the market. Identify your competitors and how your services may be different, or better – if you believe you have a USP emphasise it here. (See Chapter 5 for more on marketing.)

- *Cost analysis:* Draw up a list of anticipated costs – and double it! Include a summary of your pricing structure to show that you can balance outgoings and income in order to make a profit. (See Chapter 4 for more on calculating the start-up and ongoing costs and on pricing.)

- *Conclusion:* Reiterate your proposal, the services you wish to provide and the advantages of your business.

- *Reference list:* It is probably best to use a numerical system of referencing rather than Harvard or another system that includes names and dates. This will make your business plan easier to read, especially if it is intended for someone with no medical or academic knowledge or understanding.

- *Appendices:* Only include those that are appropriate; it is usually better to include essential information in the body of the plan rather than as an appendix.

- Appropriate appendices include a *Glossary of terms* used – for example, antenatal, frenulotomy, moxibustion, essential oils. This is important if your plan is an application for funding or to rent premises or if non-medical people will read it. It is usually preferable to use non-medical (lay) terms in the text of the plan – for example, 'moxibustion, a Chinese method to turn a breech baby to head-first', rather than 'moxibustion to avoid ECV for breech presentation'. Do not use abbreviations.

- And *your curriculum vitae* in full if you are writing the plan for a clinical setting, or a shorter biography if you are requesting funding.

Case study: Dianne Garland SRN RM ADM PGCEA MSc

MidwifeExpert (www.Midwifeexpert.com), an expert witness/legal professional reporting for solicitors and the NHS Litigation Authority.

I am an international authority/lecturer on water birth and gentle birth; a birth centre advisor for India and China; midwifery advisor to the Care Quality Commission (CQC); a governance lead for Waterbirth International; and a stakeholder for the National Institute for Health and Care Excellence (NICE) guidelines.

I started working independently in 2005, leaving my full-time NHS post as a practice development midwife. Once my business started to develop, I reduced my clinical hours and now work the equivalent of 22 hours per month, on an annualised contract, rotating in all clinical areas. My interest in expanding my skills and knowledge outside the NHS stemmed from increasing interest in and requests for legal reports and for water birth study days, and a desire to escape the oppressive culture of NHS organisations, which severely impacted on my work. I had started to put aside part of my NHS salary and all income from external work for a year before launching Midwifeexpert.com and now earn in the £20,000 to £50,000 bracket.

Your greatest achievements? Becoming known internationally, but particularly in India and China, and both developing an advisory role and enjoying the international networking.

Your biggest mistake? Under-estimating how long it can take to receive payments for work from the NHS and solicitors – it's important to have back-up finances in place.

How has your business evolved since you first started? I have recently revised my website and now have a presence on Facebook. I've further developed the various study days that I offer, worldwide. I am now at a stage when I can decide which legal cases I wish to accept. I have also been able to work with other business colleagues and companies without the constraints of the NHS.

What is the best thing about working for yourself? Being able to choose what I do each day!

What causes you most difficulty in running your own business?
Delays in being paid and then having to chase payments.

What advice would you give to a midwife/doula who is just setting out in the commercial world? Have a good website or professional Facebook page; network at every chance. Never be afraid to ask for something – the worst anyone can say is 'no'. Working for myself was the best decision I ever made – otherwise I am sure I would no longer want to work part time in a very demanding NHS.

3

Professional Issues

You may feel it is unnecessary for this book to include a section on professional issues – after all, you are already a qualified professional, you have completed appropriate training for the services you wish to offer in your new business, and you are well aware of how to act professionally. However, one of the most difficult aspects for many health professionals who move into private practice is overcoming the conflict between the caring nature of the services they provide and the commercial factors with which they must deal. This can be particularly difficult for midwives who have worked primarily in the protected environment of the NHS in which treatment for patients and clients is free at the point of access (see Chapter 4 for a discussion on charging for services). Of even more importance is the necessity to identify the boundaries of your private work and to differentiate this from any paid employment with which you may wish to continue, especially if this is in the same field as your business activities (see 'Conflicts of interest' below).

This chapter is based on the principles included in the Nursing and Midwifery Council's (NMC) document, *The Code: Professional Standards of Practice and Behaviour for Nurses and Midwives* (NMC 2015) and the codes of practice of several doula organisations, as well as Expectancy's Maternity Complementary Therapies: *Professional Code of Practice* (Tiran 2014), all of which have common themes. It is then useful to apply the principles within these codes to identify what constitutes good business practice. A midwife or doula who is professional in their approach to their work is likely to possess a personal professional philosophy that will assist in making the business a success.

In your clinical practice, the normal professional issues apply in respect of providing compassionate, safe care. Indeed, it is vital to the success of your business that you build a reputation as an empathetic and compassionate practitioner, a good listener who empowers women and involves them and their families in the decision-making process for their care and who is able to act as an advocate for them. An ability to be diplomatic, to negotiate with clients, colleagues and business associates with honesty, integrity, respect and courtesy all contributes to a dedicated sense of professionalism, which in turn boosts your unique selling point (USP). Your care and treatment of clients should focus on promoting health and wellbeing. You should explain treatments and services clearly, in terms they understand, using a range of verbal and non-verbal methods of communication; it is also necessary to check that clients have fully understood what you have discussed with them (NMC 2015, 7.1). This is particularly relevant when self-employed since not only are you totally accountable for your decisions, but any misunderstandings can lead to negative evaluations and even complaints, which may adversely affect your ability to obtain more clients.

The NMC expects you to meet the changing health needs of people (NMC 2015, 3.1). Although this is mainly intended to be interpreted in clinical terms, so that registrants are flexible in their care of patients and clients as their bio-psycho-social needs change, this could also imply a need to respond to changes in the ways healthcare is delivered. Thus, in respect of the move towards offering private services, it is appropriate to acknowledge that women are prepared to pay for services during pregnancy, birth and the puerperium – either those that are not provided by the NHS or to supplement some of those with limited availability. The nature of healthcare in general and maternity care provision in particular is changing rapidly, and you have an invaluable opportunity to be at the forefront of making some of these services available to women.

Education and training

You must, of course, be appropriately trained to provide the clinical services you wish to offer in your business. As a qualified midwife or doula you will already have undertaken the basic pre-registration training to prepare you, and it is wise to have consolidated this before setting up in private practice. At the very least, being competent and confident in your role will free up time and energy for you to learn how to set up and run your business.

However, if you wish to offer services that are not a standard component of your current role, such as complementary therapies, examination of the new-born or frenulotomy, you must be adequately and appropriately trained to provide them. This is also important if you are going to provide services that could reasonably be considered part of your existing role as a midwife or doula (see also 'Conflicts of interest', below). Defining what constitutes 'adequate and appropriate' training can be difficult, but since all health professionals must be in possession of personal professional indemnity insurance for each aspect of their work, this factor can act as a guide to accessing suitable courses. For example, a single study day on a subject such as maternity aromatherapy can only be a very basic introduction to something that is a separate professional discipline, and will not prepare you to use it, even in your NHS practice, and certainly not in private practice, without further study and maternity-related experience. If you have undertaken a short course that does not fully qualify you as an aromatherapist, you would need to use the techniques in your private practice under the umbrella qualification of your midwifery or doula work, with the relevant insurance cover. A useful benchmark for finding suitable courses is to ensure that they are directly applied to your intended services, professionally accredited, taught by suitably qualified, experienced and insured tutors and aligned to an organisation that provides successful graduates with professional indemnity insurance cover. Take care not to define 'learning' as just garnering information from colleagues in a Chinese whispers fashion without the relevant professional education from a tutor who can facilitate your application of theory to your maternity practice.

You will also need to decide how much business-related training you need to help you establish and maintain your practice (see

Chapter 2). Whilst this is not specific to the clinical services you intend to offer, being ill prepared in terms of business knowledge may impact negatively on your professional image and could, in certain circumstances, lead to issues that might bring you before a professional conduct hearing. Let us use here the example of a midwife or doula who wants to sell aromatherapy blends to her clients for which there are specific governing laws on the dispensing of medicines, both in the UK and in the European Union (EU) (NMC 2015, 18, 20.4). If you are unaware of the requirement for anyone giving or selling oil blends to be a fully qualified herbal medicine practitioner, *unless they undertake the first consultation face-to-face*, you could be found to be breaking the law. Further, there are regulations and directives governing the use of chemicals, bottling and labelling of oil blends and other issues when preparing items for sale. For midwives, and possibly also for doulas, this would then need to be reported to the regulatory body and could lead to disciplinary action, which may result in the individual being removed from the professional register.

Another more business-focused example could be that of advertising your services. There are strict rules concerning advertising, and you are not permitted to make a medical claim for your services without supporting evidence. For example, you could not guarantee to start labour in a woman wanting a post-dates pregnancy treatment – you would need to state that the treatment *may assist* in the process. In practice, it may be wise to focus on the relaxation aspect of the treatments you provide for these women, which facilitates oxytocin output. Contravening the advertising standards requirements could lead to prosecution, which again would impact on your professional registration and certainly on your business reputation (see Chapter 5 for more on marketing).

It is essential that you are aware of, and pledge to work within, the boundaries of your knowledge and training (NMC 2015, 13). It can sometimes be more difficult to maintain this in private practice because you must also consider the practice environment in which you are working. For example, following on from the example above, you may be a midwife who has trained in complementary methods to induce labour and have, perhaps, been involved in setting up a post-dates pregnancy clinic in a previous NHS post, in which you also performed membrane sweeps to aid labour onset. You may therefore consider that your training and experience are sufficient to enable you to include a membrane sweep in your post-dates pregnancy treatment in private practice. However, it is very different, in the community, from working in a hospital setting where, in the event of complications such as membrane rupture and cord prolapse, you can obtain immediate medical assistance, technological support and operating theatre access. These are not readily available to you in the community and could place you in an invidious position in the event of an emergency. In addition, you must take extra care to protect both your business and your NMC registration, so it is always wise to err on the side of caution.

Similarly, you could be a doula who has been able to work in an NHS setting, either paid as a member of staff or voluntarily. In this role you may be given more leeway to perform tasks (after training) that are not normally included in the traditional role of a doula, such as taking blood pressure recordings. In a maternity unit you have ready access to midwifery or medical practitioners who can interpret the results of your blood pressure readings and act on them quickly if necessary, but when working by yourself in the community, this would not be the case.

Your services, and the information and advice you give to women and their families, must, as always, be based on contemporary evidence (NMC 2015, 6) so that you can continue to provide safe and effective care for your clients. If you include any clinical claims on your website you must back these up with research references. Being able to discuss the latest research with clients during their consultations will set you above another practitioner providing similar services who is less well informed, and demonstrates your credibility and professionalism.

Maintaining your midwifery revalidation with the Nursing and Midwifery Council

It is essential that you undertake regular continuing professional development (CPD) pertinent both to maternity care and to any additional qualifications you may wish to use in your private practice. This is especially relevant to midwives who wish to maintain their NMC registration through revalidation (NMC 2015, 22). Ongoing professional development does not always have to be in the form of attending study days or conferences, which are costly and which take you away from your private practice, thus potentially also reducing your earnings. Learning could be in the form of reflective accounts of treatments given to pregnant or childbearing women, written reports of discussions with colleagues, reflections on professional journal papers or textbooks you have read, news items you have seen or other forms of professional development. Networking with other midwives, especially those who also provide freelance services, enables you to discuss clinical, professional and business issues that relate to the ways in which you work (see Chapter 5 on networking).

To revalidate with the NMC midwives must have completed 450 practice hours and 35 hours of CPD, including at least 20 hours of participatory learning, within the last three years. They must also submit five pieces of practice-related feedback, five written reflective accounts, a report of a reflective discussion with a confirmer, a health and character declaration and evidence of having a professional indemnity arrangement.

It can initially appear difficult to meet all the requirements for NMC revalidation, notably the 450 practice hours, especially if you have moved away from clinical practice. However, interpretation of the words 'practice hours' is wide and does not have to relate to direct *clinical* practice with hands-on care of women and babies. Midwives working as lecturers, researchers and in other settings can still count the hours of contact with 'clients' towards their revalidation; for example, the 'clients' for lecturers are the students. I have personally found this difficult since running my own company. However, as I spend all my time teaching midwives and students and can also count other activities such as revising the 9th to 13th editions of *Bailliere's Midwives' Dictionary* (see Tiran 2017), these are considered to be valid midwifery activities. It just requires a little creativity!

In your practice, you will be working directly with pregnant women, albeit probably offering services that may not be part of standard midwifery duties, but you will doubtless also be giving them information and advice, monitoring their wellbeing through your assessments prior to treatment, identifying when women need to be transferred to medical care and other aspects that fall within the remit of midwifery care. Vigilant documentation of the work you undertake with your pregnant clients can offer evidence that you are continuing to use your midwifery expertise and experience, and this will be suitable for inclusion in your required 'practice' hours. Even though you may not yet have started trading in your private practice, it can be useful to consider how you will record your practice hours. Remember, you only need the equivalent of 150 hours per year to meet the requirement of 450 practice hours for triennial revalidation with the NMC. Activity 3.1 may help you with this.

⚑ ACTIVITY 3.1: Attaining your clinical practice hours for revalidation

– Make a list of the services you intend to provide and consider the activities included within each service. Identify the amount of time you think is *directly* related to midwifery practice.

For example, if you are going to offer moxibustion as a one-hour appointment, at least half an hour of this is likely to be spent on discussing breech presentation, answering questions about other options such as external cephalic version and Caesarean section, and assessing whether the woman is suited to using moxibustion. In fact, the full hour could be counted as midwifery since you will then need to teach her and her partner how to perform the moxibustion, so this is counted as antenatal education. If you are offering antenatal classes, the entire time spent in contact with clients can be classed as midwifery, as can other services such as new-born examination, frenulotomy, lactation support or telephone advice on aspects of pregnancy.

If you work in your business just two days a week, seeing three clients a day, the number of *clinical* hours worked each week will be around six to nine (other hours will be spent on travelling and on managing your business). Taken over a 45-week year, that could potentially be between 270 and 405 hours per year of face-to-face contact, with at least half of that directly applicable to midwifery practice. If you continue to work part time as a midwife in the NHS, perhaps as a bank midwife, you will obviously count these hours as well and add any private practice hours to the total.

— Initially, however, it is likely that you will have fewer clients until you build up your business. Try to map out a possible typical working week in your new private practice, based on 30 per cent capacity (around four hours per week), which allows time for your business to build up and become established. For example, one day may include a two-hour antenatal or 'hypnobirthing' class, a 90-minute home visit to a new mother for lactation support and a one-hour relaxing massage for a pregnant woman. Whilst you may not include the full hour for the massage, you would still have here approximately four hours' worth of midwifery practice. You should now be able to calculate how much of your private practice may contribute towards your NMC practice hours requirement.

In respect of the other criteria for revalidation, it is easier to compile the evidence. The 35 hours of CPD can be in the form of courses and conferences attended, personal professional reading, attendance at journal clubs, practice-related meetings, development of clinical guidelines for your practice and other activities.

Submission of the five sets of practice-related feedback could be evaluations from clients – it is good practice anyway to invite clients to complete an evaluation form at the end of a course of treatment, and demonstrates that you are keen to provide safe, satisfying services. In marketing terms alone, there is no better advertisement than personal recommendation, and you may be able to use one or two as testimonials (with permission) on your website and literature.

For your five written reflections, these could be directly related to some of the issues that arise in your day-to-day work within your private practice.

From personal experience, I would say that the most difficult thing is making the time to write up the issues that you have faced. You may, for example, have a request from a woman for enhanced antenatal care, but you then discover that she is intending to give birth unassisted by professionals. You could discuss here the issues around 'free birthing', how you dealt with your prospective client and how you might avoid the situation arising again. A reflection can also be a discussion on something you have read in a professional journal or seen as a news item on the television. One or more of these reflective accounts can then be used as the subject of the reflective discussion with your confirmer.

Finding a confirmer may be difficult if you no longer work in the NHS. However, any senior midwife who knows you may act as your confirmer, including lecturers, mentors and line managers. You must have a face-to-face debate around your portfolio and the reflections you have recorded, and must engage in a reflective discussion with your confirmer. I have acted as a confirmer for several midwives in private practice, notably those who have completed study programmes with my company who, for various reasons, are no longer able to work in the NHS.

Activity 3.2 introduces some issues for you to reflect on. Even if you are not yet ready to start up your private practice, these could all be useful for general topics of reflection for NMC revalidation. They are also suitable for doulas who require evidence of CPD.

📌 ACTIVITY 3.2: Reflective exercises for NMC revalidation

– A client in your private practice (or a woman you see in the course of your NHS work) asks you whether she can start taking raspberry leaf tea to prepare for the labour. What do you know about raspberry leaf and how could you advise this lady? What preconceived ideas might you have that you find are challenged when you start reading about raspberry leaf? Is it safe to take it in pregnancy? Is it suitable for all women? When should women start taking it? Is there any evidence for the safety and effectiveness of raspberry leaf tea in pregnancy? Do not rely solely on what you *think* you already know – conduct a literature search and engage in some professional reading and discussions with colleagues on this subject before considering how you would answer a similar question from another woman. (See Tiran 2018, pp.233–236; you may also find the information leaflet for expectant parents, available at http://expectancy.co.uk/shop, useful for this exercise.)

— You are running an antenatal class for a group of six couples. The subject is preparation for labour. You are teaching them how to use simple massage for pain relief, and the partners are using a carrier oil to practise hand massage. One of the women suddenly starts sobbing during the session. This is a not-uncommon reaction to massage, but it can be especially difficult to deal with the situation in a group setting. What would you do and what can you learn from the experience to help you in future classes?

— You visit a new private client who is having difficulty breastfeeding her baby. During the course of your visit, you become aware of some tensions between the mother and her partner. On examination of the woman's breasts you notice some bruising and redness across her shoulders and back. When you ask her how these injuries originated, she seems evasive and uncommunicative. How would you deal with this situation and what can you learn from the experience that may have a bearing on your future midwifery or doula practice? Would you deal with this differently, dependent on whether you were working privately or in the NHS?

    — A pregnant client asks you about seeing a reflexologist to help avoid having an induction of labour. What information do you need to obtain from her and what advice should you give her to ensure she sees an appropriately trained reflexologist, and that the treatment is safe for this particular woman? What other responsibilities do you have in this situation?

Clinical competence

You must be competent and up-to-date in your practice, not only for professional purposes, but also to protect yourself against any possible claims for negligence. Your practice must be as contemporary and evidence-based as possible. Indeed, attention to detail in terms of clinical competence is perhaps even more important when working for oneself than when in the protected environment of the NHS, although the perception of protection can sometimes be misplaced. A midwifery lecturer once challenged me on this issue, stating that I could not possibly be as 'good' a lecturer now I was freelance as when I was working for the university. Perhaps this comment arose from a personal issue around asking people to pay for my services rather than providing them free at the point of access, or perhaps it was some element of professional jealousy.

In aspects of maternity care it is vital to follow a standard process from the moment of your first contact with potential clients, in your marketing and advertising (see Chapter 5), your first conversations with women and in your consultations. Comprehensive history taking is a must, recording clients' consent to treatment and perhaps a contract (see below). Irrespective of the treatment or care you provide, you will, of course, undertake a complete assessment, identifying any contraindications and precautions to the intended services.

You will need to take account of the woman's right to decline treatment and the fact that you, too, can decline to provide a service for her if you feel it is inappropriate. Deciding not to treat a woman may result in a short-term loss of income but will bring long-term gains in demonstrating that you are a professional and safe practitioner. You may wish to identify specific reasons why you would decline to treat someone, and produce a list that is available to prospective and current clients.

Table 3.1 identifies some of the reasons why you may choose not to provide your services; you may wish to add more.

Table 3.1: Reasons for declining to treat a client in your private practice

You may choose to withhold your services if any of the following situations arise:	
Medical/obstetric	General
Client has epilepsy, major cardiac, respiratory, renal or hepatic disease or is on medication for a medical or obstetric complication	Client is under the influence of alcohol or recreational drugs
Gestation inappropriate for proposed treatment	Client's, relative's or your own personal health and safety may be put at risk by the intended service, e.g., respiratory condition worsened by moxibustion, essential oils inappropriate to health of an individual
Current antepartum haemorrhage	
Placenta praevia, grades 3 or 4	
Hypertension, diastolic persistently above 85 or 90 mmHg/fulminating pre-eclampsia/history of recent eclampsia	Client has withheld information or provided false information
Twin pregnancy or higher multiples	Client is not working in partnership with you, e.g., not complying with after-care advice
Intrauterine growth retardation/abnormal fetus	Client or family member is aggressive or violent towards you
Client has active, or history of recent, carcinoma	Client or family member's words, actions or behaviour suggest that she/he is sexually attracted to you, especially if you visit the client at home
Client is not benefiting from your care	
Medical practitioner deems treatment to be inappropriate	Client is having a detrimental effect on you or your business by denigrating your professionalism or practice, verbally or in writing, in person or online
	Client is requesting services that are beyond the scope of your competence, training or insurance cover

Record keeping and data protection

All health professionals are aware that they must maintain contemporaneous, accurate and comprehensive client records that are duly signed and dated and stored safely to maintain confidentiality. In the healthcare business, this goes without saying, since you are professionally accountable for your practice. Of course, maintaining adequate records provides a protection for your client. In the event of a complaint being made against you, it may also offer an insight into your actions at the time of an incident, and could serve as a defence for you.

The Data Protection Act (2018)[1] stipulates how the records of individuals must be used and stored. Many of the requirements comply with the principles of professional record keeping for midwives and doulas, with which you will be familiar. The Act maintains that personal data (information) about people should be accurate, adequate and not excessive, up-to-date and used only for the purpose for which it is intended. The Act also states that appropriate steps must be taken to ensure that any stored data defined as 'sensitive personal material' relating to the individual's physical, mental or sexual health are not at risk of unauthorised or unlawful processing, accidental loss, damage or destruction.

Stored data relates to manual (written/paper) records maintained in an organised filing system, and to electronic records, including those kept on a desktop computer, laptop, tablet, memory stick or as audio or video recordings. Using encryption software such as BitLocker[2] may help if information is stored on your computer or you could store sensitive material in the Cloud. Individuals have the right to access their records to ensure transparency and equity. Although you may not be legally required to store your records for the 25 years relating to birth records, it may be wise to do so in case any issues arise in relation to your client, even though you may not have been directly involved. The General Data Protection Regulation (GDPR), which came into force in May 2018, aims to strengthen data protection principles for

---

1   www.legislation.gov.uk/ukpga/2018/12/contents/enacted

2   https://docs.microsoft.com/en-us/windows/security/information-protection/bitlocker/bitlocker-overview

Massage therapists (including reflexologists, shiatsu practitioners, etc.) must also hold the appropriate licence to practise, available from the local council. If you work from a centre outside your own home, you should check that the centre is licensed for these types of therapies. In some councils, both the individual and the premises must be registered, whereas other councils may not need you to register if you are a registered healthcare professional (midwife).

If you intend to play music for any treatments or in classes, you must also obtain a *music licence*, which combines both the Phonographic Performance Ltd (PPL) and Performing Rights Society (PRS) licences. This applies to *any* recorded music audible to clients and/or staff, played via the radio, television, computer, laptop or tablet, mobile telephone or any other media.[13] Even businesses that play music to people waiting on the telephone must have a PRS licence. Alternatively, you are permitted to use royalty-free music – and there are many sources of specific relaxation music that are copyright-free. If the woman listens to her own music via a mobile telephone or iPod this is acceptable, but should not be publicly audible.

Health and safety law must be complied with, both for yourself and any employees, but also to protect women and their families visiting you, in whatever setting you may work in. Health and safety law applies to anyone, whether self-employed or not, whose work poses a threat to the health and/or safety of others. Identify possible risks and take steps to minimise them. This might involve the use of chemicals such as aromatherapy oils, equipment including examination or therapy couches and chairs, needles used for acupuncture, or any electrical equipment used in the course of your work.

Non-disclosure agreements may be appropriate in certain circumstances. These are written agreements that ensure confidentiality relating to shared information, even with suppliers of equipment or goods to support your business. The more confidential information your business plan contains, the more important these agreements become. Non-disclosure agreements do not, however, relate to client records that are protected under the GDPR (see above).

---

13   www.gov.uk/licences-to-play-background-music

all individuals within the European Union (EU). Fines are imposed for breaches of data protection, which, in extreme circumstances, could be as much as £500,000.

Box 3.1 summarises aspects of record keeping relating to data protection.

Box 3.1: Record keeping for data protection

- *All* aspects of treatment, advice given verbally or in writing, products or equipment used must be recorded comprehensively, contemporaneously, legibly and in English (or in the official language of the country in which you work).

- All consultations, including follow-up appointments, face-to-face, telephone or Skype consultations, must be recorded, signed and dated.

- Client information obtained and kept on record must be relevant to the treatment and care and should not be excessive.

- Clients must be made aware of the purpose of any records you keep and how they will be used.

- It is recommended that the absence of significant issues is recorded fully to indicate that you have fully assessed the client; for example, rather than recording 'no contraindications', it is preferable to record 'no vaginal bleeding, no hypertension, no oedema present', etc., which demonstrates that you have given thought to the potential for their occurrence.

- Full information regarding any anticipated effects of treatment or care, both positive and negative, including potential healing reactions, should be discussed and a record made that the client has confirmed her understanding of this discussion.

- In the event of adverse reactions occurring, a record should be made of the symptoms, advice and/or care given to deal with them and any referral to medical care.

- Client evaluations of treatment should be recorded, including informal verbal responses.

- Most insurers require clinical records to be kept for a minimum of ten years. However, where care is provided that is specific midwifery care or advice, or when caring for a woman in labour, in any capacity, records should be kept for the mandatory 25 years to comply with the Civil Liabilities Act (1978).

- In the event of the need to refer for medical or standard midwifery care, written permission of the client must be obtained and any records, or copies of records, which are passed to other practitioners must remain confidential.

- All clients have the right to access their records.

- All records containing personal data from which an individual can be identified must be stored securely (consider software such as BitLocker for Windows 10, which allows encryption of sensitive data).

- Any business processing personal data on a computer, including obtaining, recording, using, storing and disclosing information, must be registered with the Information Commissioner's Office (ICO).

Professional image

Portraying a professional image and demeanour is crucial to avoid compromising the integrity of your business. A professional image centres round the characteristics and qualities that reflect your competence, confidence and character as judged by your clients and associates. This may include qualities such as integrity, trustworthiness, commitment, being caring and capable.

Whilst you may have specific ideas about how you wish to appear to your clients, you must also take into account the fact that your practice is based on midwifery or doula qualifications, and that there is therefore an expectation pertinent to all healthcare professionals. Developing a professional image means considering how you look, your body and verbal language, your attitudes and behaviour and the ways in which you communicate with clients, colleagues and business associates.

First impressions are critical and can be made within a few seconds of meeting you – you never get a chance to make another *first* impression. Decide what you want to be and how you wish to present yourself to your clients. Is it important to you to be business-like, informal, stylish or 'cool'? Can you reconcile your choices with being both a healthcare professional and a businessperson?

Although it is not necessary to have a uniform, clothing appropriate to your practice is necessary, but this may differ according to what you do and the clients with whom you are working. Businesspeople often 'dress for success', but this may imply something more formal than you wish to portray or than will suit your clients. If you are providing manual treatments you will need to be comfortable yet smart, so perhaps trousers with a polo or t-shirt appeals to you.

I find dressing for my business particularly difficult because I want to be informal enough to be on a par with midwives and doulas who are my prospective students, yet smart enough, especially when in a maternity unit, to appear professional if I meet senior personnel. I tend to wear trousers because I may be on the floor demonstrating massage or positions for labour, and I have developed a sort of 'uniform' of black trousers and top with a smart jacket over them that I can remove when teaching practical skills. I also travel a lot so I have to consider how well everything packs, and tend to buy clothes that crush up well and can be hand-washed and drip-dried without the need for ironing (I usually try to take only hand luggage to avoid the risk of cases being lost, as happened the first time I went to teach in Japan!).

You may also wish to have a name badge or to mount a business card on a lanyard to show to clients, particularly when visiting women in their own homes. Any equipment you use, or the bags in which you carry the tools of your trade, need to be neat, clean and in keeping with the overall image of your business. You can claim tax relief on clothing and other items used *solely and exclusively* for work purposes (they may need to have a logo on them to identify them as being for business use).

Your attitude goes a long way towards making clients feel comfortable with you. Using positive body language that shows confidence, professionalism and trust, without being intimidating, is good for business too. You may feel incredibly nervous when you first start seeing private clients but try not to show it. If you feel comfortable with it, shake hands when you meet people – although not all your clients will offer their hands, many business contacts will do so. Concentrate on your clients, however pressurised you feel – you no longer have the excuse of a busy maternity unit behind which you can hide! If your clients feel that your mind is on something else whilst talking to them, they may decline your services and possibly post negative comments on social media.

In relation to your online presence, set up a separate Facebook page or Instagram account for your business, and keep it solely for advertising, adding news, testimonials and photographs (with permission) that are directly related to your business. In addition, take care what you post on your personal social media – clients may not wish to see you inebriated at someone's party! If possible, clean up your personal pages and remove anything that may have a detrimental effect on your business, and ask your friends to do the same. Although not related to private practice, I know of a midwife whose friend in Australia posted information about her at a time when the midwife was sick, yet her manager saw the post and mistakenly assumed that the midwife had actually been on holiday in Australia whilst claiming illness. Social media can be your friend or your enemy – and no more so than when you have your own business (see NMC 2017 for the NMC's guidance on the use of social media, which could apply equally to doulas).

Decide how formal you will be when interacting with clients, especially when communicating by email or text. Avoid starting your emails with 'Hi', at least in the first instance, and *never* when the email subject concerns money or legal issues or when you are communicating with other clinical professionals. Avoid using 'x' (kisses) at the end of your emails and identify a professional signature in keeping with your personal philosophy. Even though you may want to be relaxed when working with clients, not everyone wishes to do the same. Some clients can feel uncomfortable with enforced informality or familiarity or conversely, by too formal an approach. The skill is to assess your clients and to act accordingly.

You even need to think about your car if you are visiting women in their own homes. It should be clean and well maintained. It will not be pleasant if you need a new exhaust fitting and the car emits smoke and is excessively noisy when you arrive or leave the house. If you decide to have a logo on the car it must be adhered properly (and straight!), and it may be better to ask a professional to do this for you.

Whilst much of this section will not be new to you, and you may even feel it is superfluous to your needs when you are busy developing your business, it is important to your ultimate success. Being aware of who you are and how others perceive you will help you to develop a professional profile that will set you aside from others through a sense of self-belief and self-worth. It is vital to be remembered for the right reasons, not those that are likely to detract from your business success.

Activity 3.3 is designed to help you become more aware in terms of preparing for your business. It can be surprising to reflect on the image you portray to others – it may not be quite what you think!

ACTIVITY 3.3: Developing your professional image for business

    – How would you like your clients to see you? What image are you trying to offer to (a) your clients, (b) your colleagues and (c) your business associates? You may want to ask a colleague or friend to give you an honest opinion about the ways in which other people see you.

    – What might your clients, colleagues and business associates say about you when you are absent? Identify any aspects of your desired professional image on which you may need to work for improvement.

— Think about the specifics – What will you wear? How will your clients view your car? Are the items you need for consultations logically and neatly organised? Are you familiar with the consultation forms you will be using, either in hard copy or digital form?

Contracts between yourself and your clients

A contract is an agreement between you and your client and sets out the expectations of both the practitioner and client – emphasising that you both have rights and responsibilities in the interaction between you.

From a professional viewpoint, you must provide potential and actual clients with visible, easy-to-understand information on any fees and charging policies. This is also good business practice. The information you provide should include points such as charges for cancellations, missed appointments, methods of payment and the scheduling of and requirements for any payments by instalment (see Chapter 4 on charging). If appropriate, you should also make clear the arrangements for any back-up provision in the event of you being unable to provide the services for which a woman has paid (if you are unwell, on holiday or called up for jury service, for example).

It can be helpful to negotiate a contract with your clients, especially if you are providing care over a period of time, for example, ongoing doula support services from pregnancy through to the postnatal period or a course of complementary therapy treatments during pregnancy. This emphasises the need to work in partnership with women, but also reinforces the fact that 'a partnership' is a two-way affair that requires some commitment from the woman. A contract not only relates to issues around payment; it may also include essential clinical aspects, for example, gaining explicit consent to treatment after providing the woman with sufficient information so that she can make informed choices. You may wish to include the fact that *you* have the right to decline to treat a woman in the event that you feel what she is requesting is inappropriate or untimely (see above).

A contract should be written in formal language; use a standard format that can be adapted to each client as necessary. You may prefer to use the services of a solicitor to help you with this. Box 3.2 lists the issues you may wish to include in your contract.

Box 3.2: The client–practitioner contract

You may wish to include some or all of the following clauses in a contract with your clients:

- Explanation of what you will provide for the client and what service she can expect from you.

- Definition of the services you will not provide – for example, you will not agree to conduct a 'natural induction' treatment before at least 37 weeks' gestation.

- Requirement for the client to bring her standard maternity 'handheld' notes with her to each appointment – this ensures she is not opting for unassisted birth and enables you to read the notes for background information (although you may not write in them).

- Acknowledgement that the information the client provides is accurate and truthful.

- A request that clients arrive punctually – and your policy if they arrive late; it is normal to shorten the duration of the appointment so that you can finish on time for your next scheduled client.

- Duration and venue of the appointment, and course of treatment if relevant.

- How clients may contact you, as well as an agreement about when you should not be contacted (unless in an emergency, if relevant to your services).

- What the client can expect in relation to data protection and maintenance of client records, including confidentiality and consent.

- What the client can expect in terms of clear sexual boundaries and gender equality.

- Asking the client's permission to refer to other practitioners, in particular the client's midwife, general practitioner (GP) or obstetrician, if her condition requires it.

- Cancellations, postponements, forgotten appointments – payment and rearranging appointments.

- Your fees and the required method(s) of payment – for example, payment in advance or in instalments.

- Add any other issues you would wish a contract to address.

Conflicts of interest

One of the most difficult issues for midwives and doulas to deal with is that of conflicts of interest. This may be a conflict between your clinical and business roles, a difference between your midwifery/doula role and that of the services you provide in a self-employed capacity, or a conflict between being an NHS employee and also working in private practice.

A joint statement on this latter issue was published in February 2017 by NHS England,[3] which set out certain principles and rules for identifying, avoiding, minimising and managing conflicts of interest. This was followed in August 2017 by a statement from the NMC[4] that was specific to NMC registrants, and the principles refer to all four countries of the UK. Other Royal Colleges have also published statements relevant to their own registrants. The NHS England statement refers only to NHS employees, so if you do not work within the NHS, you are not bound by its requirements, although the principles pertain, in general terms, to all private practitioners, particularly those with a statutory registration such as midwives.

It was acknowledged by all parties involved in devising the joint statement that conflicts can arise in situations where a practitioner's judgement may be influenced by a personal, financial or other interest, particularly when it involves people working in complex systems such as the NHS. 'Interests' may be defined as directly financial or as personal or professional non-financial benefits (such as promises of career promotion) or indirect benefits. The joint statement emphasised

---

3   www.england.nhs.uk/ourwork/coi
4   www.nmc.org.uk/news/news-and-updates/conflicts-of-interest-joint-statement

that the NHS commitments of all its staff must take precedence over private practice. One suggestion was made that doctors, dentists and others should be required to publish details of their income from work undertaken outside the NHS. The Royal College of Surgeons (2016) opposed this, claiming that is it not relevant and that a requirement to do so implies that the NHS 'does not trust' its staff.[5] At the time of writing this suggestion has, thankfully, not been implemented.

You must declare any existing work in which you engage outside your NHS employment, and steps may be considered by managers in order to reduce the risk of conflict. You may be required to seek approval *prior* to working in private practice, and must declare the nature, dates and duration of your outside work, once commenced. If you believe that a conflict of interest has arisen or is likely to arise, you should formally notify your manager, in writing. You are not, in any circumstances, permitted to promote your private practice whilst engaged in NHS activities, nor should you ask other staff to initiate such discussions on your behalf. You are also required to declare non-clinical roles you may hold outside your NHS employment, such as consultancy work or acting as a charity trustee or school governor. If you are paid to present a paper at a conference you must now also declare this, even if you choose to donate your fee to a charitable organisation.

Many of the issues raised by the NMC's statement on conflicts of interest are similar to clauses contained in *The Code* (NMC 2015), and the statement is intended to be used in conjunction with *The Code*. For example, the maintenance of appropriate personal and professional boundaries with clients and their families is fundamental to good professional practice. These can, however, be difficult to maintain, particularly when working alone and in a non-clinical environment such as the mother's own home, since many of the traditional boundaries have been eroded, and the interaction between healthcare practitioners and their clients is more informal and relaxed. You must also ensure that your professional judgement is not compromised by commercial interests or incentives, such as payment for using particular

5   www.rcseng.ac.uk/news-and-events/media-centre/press-releases/statement-on-conflicts-of-interest-and-private-practice

products in your practice. You must refuse expensive gifts or favours, the acceptance of which could contravene your code of practice.

A midwife colleague of mine who was just setting out on her journey to work in private practice offering breastfeeding support, acupuncture, moxibustion and treatment for post-dates pregnancy, was challenged by her midwifery manager about her involvement in a local breastfeeding support group, which she had joined to supplement her own learning. The manager informed her that she was not eligible to become a member of the group as she was neither a new mother nor an expert in lactation support. When, during the conversation, the midwife also informed her that she was intending to offer various services privately, the manager erroneously stated that the midwife must inform the NMC. You are not, however, required to notify the NMC that you are working privately. You are an autonomous practitioner registered to provide the services for which you are trained; for midwives this does not mean that you are committed to working solely in the NHS, and there should be nothing in your NHS contract that prevents you from doing so. The somewhat draconian requirements of NHS England's statement seem to have caused greater confusion amongst some NHS personnel than even before it was published.

There is also the issue of antagonism from managers and other midwives working solely in the NHS. Unfortunately, many NHS staff remain ill disposed towards clinicians offering private services (this has long been seen in relation to medical consultants who work privately in addition to their NHS contracts). However, this does not appear to be in sympathy with the issue of choice for women who may want to pay for certain services. One of the tenets of contemporary maternity care is the need to offer women more choice in the way they receive their maternity care. Indeed, the Personal Maternity Care Budget (PMCB) is designed for this purpose. Further, it does not take account of the fact that midwives (and other staff) have choices in the way they work, including whether to remain practising solely in the NHS, to work as independent midwives or to offer other maternity-related services for which woman pay. It is therefore unacceptable that managers and others denigrate midwives who are far-sighted enough to appreciate that women actually want these services. I frequently receive telephone calls from midwives who have chosen to work in private practice part time alongside their NHS work, but who are experiencing hostility from colleagues.

You must be extremely careful to recognise the boundaries between those aspects of your work that are deemed to be 'true midwifery' and those that are not. This applies equally to doulas as to midwives. 'Midwifery' aspects would include those practices that are legally defined as being within the role of a midwife, particularly when taking sole responsibility for birth services. If you choose to offer antenatal and postnatal care, you should not undertake any aspects of care with your private clients that could be construed as part of midwifery practice unless you are also in possession of the necessary indemnity insurance cover (see below). Issues can arise in which you feel compelled to undertake something from a point of view of safety, but which might be interpreted as a midwifery task.

An example here is your decision to undertake an abdominal examination to confirm fetal presentation prior to teaching a woman how to perform moxibustion for breech presentation. If a woman consulted an acupuncturist for moxibustion, abdominal examination would not be performed since it is not part of the practitioner's remit, but she would be assessed in different ways to ensure the suitability of treatment. Conversely, as a midwife, if you failed to perform the abdominal examination this could be seen as negligent if complications arise which might have been avoided with adequate obstetric assessment, for example, cephalopelvic disproportion resulting in obstruction.

For midwives working privately whilst continuing to work as employed midwives for the NHS, obvious potential conflicts relate to financial interests. It is therefore essential that you put the interests of clients first, both in terms of clinical considerations and their vulnerability when choosing to pay for services. You must be able to assess your clients in order to determine whether or not it is appropriate to provide them with the services they are requesting, and feel able to decline to treat them, if necessary (see above). You should not, for example, suggest that you can provide a course of treatment that is not clinically relevant, merely to increase your income. This goes without saying but can sometimes be easy to forget when you may be focused on the need to make money to earn a living.

A way of protecting yourself from many of the potential areas for conflict is to devise guidelines for your practice that state clearly the women you will treat and those you will not. These guidelines can then be made available to your potential clients, on your website, in your clinic room or in a folder that you offer if working peripatetically. Using the example of a woman requesting moxibustion, it would be contraindicated if she has a previous Caesarean section scar on the uterus that is less than two years old. Should you agree to treat her you would be working outside the accepted parameters for midwives providing moxibustion. Showing her your practice guidelines would reinforce the point to her that your decision is based on standard practice. You could advise her to pursue an alternative option and consult a qualified acupuncturist who would take responsibility for her treatment. This is not so much a case of 'passing the buck', but would mean that a more experienced professional, who is able to assess the woman in terms of traditional Chinese medicine principles rather than obstetrically, would assume responsibility for the treatment under their own therapy insurance.

Conversely, it may sometimes be appropriate for you to compromise by offering alternative services to the ones the woman may be requesting, because this is in her best interests, in accordance with the NMC *Code* (2015). An increasingly common example is that of a woman wanting treatment for post-dates pregnancy, in terms of 'natural induction of labour'. You may deduce from your assessment that she is clinically unsuited to the treatment, perhaps because she has not yet reached term or has a complicated pregnancy. Offering to provide some gentle relaxation treatment so that you can spend time with her, answering questions and working to reduce her cortisol levels to facilitate natural oxytocin release, may be better than declining to treat her at all. A decision not to treat could result in her choosing to consult a complementary practitioner who may not fully understand the clinical issues. Indeed, I know of a reflexology clinic, currently under scrutiny from the relevant regulatory organisations, where therapists agree to perform specific treatments to trigger contractions – without taking a history, looking at the woman's maternity records or making any record of the treatment. They rely on the woman to inform them of the gestation and do not seem to have any understanding of the potential dangers of inappropriate treatment (personal communications with national regulatory organisations).

If you are employed by the NHS or any other organisation, whether in healthcare or not, you must avoid using *any* time or facilities in your workplace that relate to your business. For example, you cannot answer telephone calls from prospective clients whilst in your place of employment nor use the photocopier to copy leaflets for them – this would be considered stealing, and is usually a reason for dismissal. This applies equally to those whose employed work is in a designated building such as a maternity unit, and to those who work peripatetically including community-based midwives or support workers or doulas who are employed by an organisation.

Activity 3.4 provides some clinical scenarios that you may wish to consider in relation to conflicts of interest. These exercises could also be used towards NMC revalidation.

ACTIVITY 3.4: Clinical scenarios of conflicts of interest

You are continuing to work as a midwife in your local unit. You are not permitted to advertise your services overtly to the women in your care, but may have been given permission to leave your leaflets in the antenatal clinic. Here are some scenarios that may occur. How would you deal with them?

- A woman telephones for information on your private antenatal classes, which she has seen advertised in the local community magazine. You realise that she is one of the expectant mothers in your own team's caseload. How would you deal with this? Is it acceptable to agree to treat her privately?

– An expectant mother comes to your private practice for acupuncture for backache and pelvic girdle pain at 35 weeks' gestation. During your assessment she reports that she has a headache and you note that she has very oedematous ankles. You ask her some pertinent questions and she tells you she has had flashing lights before her eyes. You conclude that she may have severe pre-eclampsia. How would you deal with this situation? Would you actually take her blood pressure? Would you treat her in the hope that the relaxation aspects of your treatment may bring her blood pressure down? What are your responsibilities in this case?

– You are at work in the NHS maternity unit and you see a woman in the antenatal clinic who asks you if you know anyone who provides treatment for 'natural induction' of labour (which you provide in your private services). How would you deal with this situation? Is it acceptable to give her your leaflets? If you do not provide a service for her, what are the chances that she may go elsewhere, perhaps to someone who is less well trained than you? What are the professional, legal and ethical issues here?

Disclosure and Barring Service checks

The Disclosure and Barring Service (DBS) is part of the UK Home Office services, formed in 2012 when the Criminal Records Bureau (CRB) and the Independent Safeguarding Authority (ISA)[6] were merged under the Protection of Freedoms Act 2012.[7] It was established to ensure protection for vulnerable people by checking the credentials of people applying to work with children, people with mental ill health or with a disability, and other susceptible adults. Potential employees undergo a check through the Police National Computer to determine whether they have a criminal record. A basic check will disclose any cautions, reprimands, warnings and convictions deemed to be unspent according to the Rehabilitation of Offenders Act 1974.[8] A standard check is similar but an enhanced check is usually undertaken for those seeking posts with high levels of responsibility. The enhanced check relates to healthcare professionals, teachers and others if the applicant's job role is specified in both the Rehabilitation of Offenders Act 1974 (Exception) Order 1975 and the Police Act 1997. This latter category includes midwives employed by the NHS or an independent organisation.

Most midwives who have recently worked in the NHS are likely to be in possession of a current certificate showing that they are not barred from working with mothers and babies. Since 2013, the certificates have been considered portable between employers. If you do not have a copy of your DBS/original CRB check because you have been in your current post since before 2013, you may be able to ask your employer for a copy. Old CRB certificates remain valid in law, although in reality they become out-dated as soon as they are issued since someone could commit a crime the very next day, which might lead to them being barred from working with vulnerable people.

It is not a legal requirement to have a DBS certificate if you are self-employed, although it is, of course, a serious offence to seek to work with vulnerable children and adults after having been barred from doing so. It may, however, be reassuring to be able to

---

6   https://en.wikipedia.org/wiki/Independent_Safeguarding_Authority
7   https://en.wikipedia.org/wiki/Protection_of_Freedoms_Act_2012
8   https://en.wikipedia.org/wiki/Rehabilitation_of_Offenders_Act_1974

tell prospective clients that you have been cleared to work with families. This information could also be included on your website and marketing leaflets. If you do not have a DBS certificate – and this may include doulas – you can submit a Subject Access Request to your local police force that can provide you with a certificate containing similar information to the DBS certificate (for a fee). Local arrangements for obtaining an application form can vary between regions, so it may be easiest to telephone your local police and ask to speak to the Data Protection team. To complete the application form you will need two forms of identification, one with your name and a photograph, for example, a driving licence, and the other with your current address, such as a utility bill or bank statement, plus the relevant fee. This will be a basic check; only a prospective employer can apply for a standard or enhanced check. You could also approach your local council to undertake a DBS check for you. If you have formed a limited company you are not technically self-employed and may be able to request DBS checks for your 'staff' (i.e., yourself).

Insurance

All healthcare professionals are required by law to be in possession of *professional indemnity insurance* to protect them against claims for medical negligence or malpractice. You must be fully cognisant of the parameters of your indemnity insurance policy and not undertake any practice for which you are not covered. You must also inform your insurance provider of any change in your personal circumstances that may have a bearing on your policy cover. When embarking on new training courses it is wise to check whether completion of the course entitles you to obtain indemnity insurance cover to use it in your private practice. Documents relating to your insurance must be available in the event of a client requesting confirmation of your cover. You would also be wise to include brief details of your insurance cover on your website and other marketing materials, such as the organisation with which you are insured and your policy number.

Depending on the services you offer, you may need more than one source of indemnity insurance cover. You may, for example, have trained in a particular complementary therapy and have insurance as a full practitioner for that, but may also wish to provide other maternity services that are not covered by the same organisation. It can be expensive to have several insurance policies, so it is wise to search for the one that covers you for most of the services you offer and then take out any extra insurance for other practices. An example of this might be a doula who is trained in aromatherapy, reflexology and 'hypnobirthing'. It is likely that training for each discipline will be aligned to a specific organisation, but the doula will not then be covered for doula services or antenatal education. It may therefore be more cost-effective to register with a broader organisation that provides cover for all aspects of maternity work (as opposed to general therapy work), such as the Federation of Antenatal Educators (FEDANT).[9]

Midwives working in private practice will not be adequately covered by membership with the Royal College of Midwives (RCM). RCM indemnity insurance covers you only for 'occasional' private work, which is undefined but generally taken to refer to caring for a friend in labour or undertaking significantly less private work than NHS practice. The Royal College of Nursing (RCN) will, however, cover you for private antenatal and postnatal care, maternity complementary therapies and antenatal education. It will not cover you for any service involving incisions, such as circumcision or frenulotomy, nor will it permit the use of homeopathy or, somewhat inexplicably, lactation consultancy (although this latter can be construed as antenatal and postnatal education). On the other hand, some issues are open to interpretation. For example, you could question whether it is essential to hold insurance cover for something such as baby massage if you are already insured for general massage. Similarly, it is not possible to obtain indemnity insurance for moxibustion for breech presentation unless you are a fully qualified – and insured – acupuncturist, but if you teach expectant parents how to perform this technique for themselves, it can be considered under the umbrella term of 'antenatal education'.

At the time of writing, there is no cover for midwives wishing to provide birth services for women because the cost of insuring them for high-risk intrapartum care is prohibitive. Independent Midwives UK (IM UK) challenged this in 2017, arguing that denying midwives the

9   www.fedant.org

right to work independently diminished choice of place of birth for women and choice of work environments for midwives. In protecting the public, the High Court upheld the decision of the NMC that indemnity insurance arrangements in place at that time did not provide adequate cover for private midwives attending women in labour, as it would be insufficient to meet a claim for catastrophic injury such as cerebral palsy.[10] More recently, some independent midwives have negotiated honorary or bank contracts with NHS trusts prepared to insure them under the trust's vicarious liability cover (see the RCN's advice on self-employment[11]). The RCM's website does not provide comprehensive information on working for oneself, and most of their coverage relates to independent midwifery including the provision of birth services.[12]

Public liability (PL) insurance is optional but recommended if you decide to buy or rent premises, for example, to set up your own clinic. It is morally essential when interacting with members of the public. Even if you choose to work from your own home, it may be wise to take out PL insurance to protect you and your clients (and their partners or children) who visit you. PL insurance covers the buildings you use for your practice, and protects you from expensive lawsuits if someone is injured, for example, a client falling over your doorstep and breaking a leg, or getting caught on a loose nail, causing a scratch that then becomes seriously infected, necessitating time off work. PL insurance also protects you if you visit women in their own homes and inadvertently cause damage to their property, for instance, spilling massage oil on a precious rug or computer. The policy will normally cover you to resolve the issue and for any legal fees incurred in settling disputes. If you rent rooms in a clinic, the organisation to which you pay rental fees should have PL insurance – and when looking for suitable premises you should enquire about this. PL cover may be included with your indemnity insurance if you decide to operate as a sole trader.

---

10 www.nmc.org.uk/registration/staying-on-the-register/professional-indemnity-arrangement

11 www.rcn.org.uk/get-help/rcn-advice/self-employment

12 www.rcm.org.uk/content/independent-midwives-faqa

Product liability insurance is required if you intend to produce or sell goods. You have a duty of care to provide your clients with written information on how to use the products and any risks associated with proper use of the products and the dangers of incorrect or inappropriate use. If you intend to *dispense* herbal, homeopathic or Bach flower remedies or essential oils, you are legally required to have specific dispensing qualifications and insurance according to EU regulations that came into force in April 2011. You may be wise only to *advise* women on natural remedies and direct them to a suitable source from which they can purchase the remedies themselves. This does not currently apply to oils etc. that you use during the course of an appointment, but any oil remaining from a treatment you have given and that you then give (or sell) to the mother for use at home should be clearly and adequately labelled, and a leaflet with more in-depth information about correct usage should also be given. You are not permitted to blend oils and give them or sell them to women unless you have done the first treatment with the same blend. It is, however, permissible to keep a small stock of remedies produced commercially to sell or give to women so that they can begin their treatment straight away, although you must remember to adhere to medicines law and guidelines, especially if you are a midwife retaining your registration with the NMC.

Other insurance policies that you will need to check include your household contents and building insurance if you work from home and your motor vehicle insurance if you drive to clients' homes. Failure to clarify these policies may invalidate them in the event of a claim needing to be made. You may also wish to investigate whether it is worth taking out insurance against your inability to work though illness or injury and private health insurance to cover you for prompt access to treatment to enable you to take minimal time away from your business. *Protected income insurance* provides cover for other reasons why you may not be able to work, for example, jury service, and may be wise if your business is your only source of income. *Employers' insurance* is legally required if you employ one or more people in your business. It covers the costs of any compensation payable to employees in the event of a work-related injury or illness. Activity 3.5 will help you identify your insurance requirements.

☝ ACTIVITY 3.5: Identifying your insurance requirements

- Make a list of the types of insurance cover you will need for your proposed business, based on the information above and any other issues you have identified.

- Do some online research to help you estimate how much this will cost you each year. If you already have insurance, for example, with the Royal College of Midwives or Doula UK, you should count this in your total costs of insurance, as this now becomes a legitimate business expense, even though you were previously paying this yourself.

Legal issues

It is essential, when setting up a business, to ensure that you are aware of the legal aspects involved. The first, and most important issue in the early days, is to determine the *structure* of your business (see Chapter 2).

You may need to apply for a *licence*, especially if you intend to work from home. In England, Wales and Northern Ireland, if you are going to practise acupuncture you must register with your local authority as a 'skin piercer', and your premises and hygiene standards could be liable to inspection. In Greater London the regulations differ and acupuncturists who are not registered with a statutorily regulated profession (midwife, nurse, doctor) must hold a licence that is renewed annually. In Scotland, all acupuncture practitioners must be licensed.

Sale of products

'Conflicts of interest' also applies to the production of goods as well as clinical services. It is perfectly acceptable to sell products that have been commercially produced and that comply with the various legal regulations relevant to the product. However, there appears to be a growing number of midwives who are developing their own products to sell to clients. This includes educational materials, applications and notably, aromatherapy oil blends, candles or soaps. There are numerous UK and EU regulations governing medicines, chemicals and production of goods relating to health and safety, especially hygiene, labelling, fire prevention, use of glass bottles and many other issues. It is not the purpose of this book to provide comprehensive information on production of items for sale, but if this is something you wish to do, you must investigate thoroughly before making a start.

For the Aromatherapy Trade Council's (ATC) information on the legalities of making aromatherapy oil blends, see ATC (2011); you should also investigate the Cosmetics Regulations for more on this.[14] The British Candlemakers Association offers guidance on the production and sale of aromatic candles.[15] Educational materials must comply with intellectual copyright laws.[16]

Dealing with complaints

Of course, you will endeavour to provide the best service possible, and the relationship you have with your clients will generally mean that any minor dissatisfactions can be dealt with promptly and diplomatically. However, as your business grows, you will not be able to please all your clients all the time and complaints do sometimes arise. In almost 15 years I have only ever had two formal complaints, both from midwives who felt aggrieved at the academic marks they had received (fail grades), and the fact that this would not therefore

14 www.businesscompanion.info/en/quick-guides/product-safety/cosmetic-products

15 www.britishcandles.org/documents/www.britishcandles.org/Trading_Standards/candlesadvicesheet(v5).pdf

16 www.gov.uk/government/publications/notice-34-intellectual-property-rights/notice-34-intellectual-property-rights   and   https://ico.org.uk/media/for-organisations/documents/1632/eir_intellectual_property_rights.pdf

permit them to work in private practice. Both these individuals lacked the self-awareness to acknowledge their own faults, which made them angry and disappointed in the outcomes. Fortunately, my company has robust policies and procedures in place, including academic regulations and a formal complaints process, which enabled us to deal with both complaints and to revise our documents to take account of potential new issues arising.

Obtaining evaluations from your clients, either verbally or in writing, can often reduce the likelihood of minor dissatisfactions becoming formal complaints, and you should act on any issue that is raised repeatedly by clients. It is important to deal with informal and formal complaints professionally, and you must not allow them to influence negatively the ongoing care you provide. If you feel that the complaint adversely affects the relationship you have with the client, it may be wise to find another practitioner to take over the care or to discontinue the care (if clinically appropriate) and offer a refund of any fees already paid. You should try to learn from complaints, reflect on them and use them to improve your practice or the way in which your business is organised. You should also try not to take them personally, although this can be very hard – after all, this is *your* business and it is natural that you will see any negative comments as a complaint against *you*, but this is not normally the case.

Case study: Sarah Bryan LLB (Hons) B Mid (Hons) RM Cert Ed

Sarah Bryan Private Midwifery (www.sarahbryanprivatemidwifery.co.uk or www.sarahbryan.co.uk), based in Central South England and the Thames Valley, offering enhanced midwifery services, and complementary therapies including clinical hypnosis, and antenatal classes.

Whilst practising as an NHS midwife, I had already begun to lay the foundations towards independent midwifery. Spinal injury brought an abrupt end to my NHS career, but it was the catalyst to undertaking further training with Expectancy and establishing my own business as an independent midwife and practitioner of midwifery complementary therapies. I wanted to create space for nurturing the physical, emotional and mental wellbeing of mothers and babies. By utilising traditional midwifery skills, complementary therapies, my experience as a doula and Active Birth yoga teacher, and my knowledge gained through postgraduate research, my practice aims to balance the science and art of midwifery within a holistic framework.

Your greatest achievements? I was able to secure with ease a small 'start-up' loan that is well supported by the government for small businesses. I also borrowed some money from a family member and was able to avoid some set-up costs by undertaking much of the legwork myself, such as building a website.

How has your business evolved since you first started? Although I have previously worked as a private doula and antenatal teacher, my current business has only just begun, and I am looking forward to developing it and growing with it.

What is the best thing about working for yourself? The ability to prioritise family and personal life alongside work commitments, rather than the demands of work dominating everything! Professionally, it is the opportunity to practise with true autonomy and the ability to take time with clients and offer the 'gold standard' of care. Every aspect of midwifery practice becomes more authentic and integral.

What causes you most difficulty in running your own business? Dealing with potential conflicts of interest around professional boundaries and which 'hat' I am wearing. As a midwife, the 'world of business' has been overwhelming at times as there is so much to learn. Setting up the website, attaching a price tag to my services and then marketing them, networking, and managing all the 'extras' like expenses and accounts have certainly required guidance and support. I have also faced personal challenges around my self-belief and self-compassion, learning to nurture myself rather than being in a battle with the demands of life/work.

What advice would you give to a midwife/doula who is just setting out in the commercial world? It is important that we, as midwives, do not under-estimate the magnitude of our purpose. Whilst I have acknowledged some reluctance to charge for my services, the NHS maternity services are crumbling, and a new way forward must be forged, both professionally and culturally. Women are prepared to pay for what they want for this huge life event of pregnancy and birth, and we are there to provide it for them.

4

Financial Issues

It is vital to get to grips with the financial aspects of setting up and maintaining your business. After all, this may be the only source of income for you. However, perhaps for the first time ever, you will be dealing with *paying customers* face-to-face. It can be difficult for those of us in the caring professions to become familiar with the intricacies of setting prices, sorting out budgets, dealing with Her Majesty's Revenue & Customs (HMRC, formerly the Inland Revenue), and keeping accounts records. From personal experience I can tell you it is very daunting and even now, every time an unanticipated letter arrives from HMRC, I go into panic mode and frantically contact my accountant!

You need to consider some financial basics, particularly if you are intending to work in your practice full time and are giving up the 'day job', the work that has automatically provided you with a regular and stable income. In the beginning you may want to continue working in your current post and perhaps even plan to save towards setting up your business. There will, however, come a time when you just have to take that plunge and commit fully to your new venture. There is nothing like 'feeling hungry' or having financial commitments at home to motivate you to do well in your business, but you must also use your common sense and look at your personal circumstances. If you have someone else at home who is earning, it may be a little easier for you to take some time to build up your business without being too financially compromised, but if you are doing this on your own, you may need to delve into savings, or even apply for a loan to fund your first few months.

Consider how much income you need to live on – and what you would like to earn in order to maintain your standard of living. How does this compare with the amount of work you need to do to achieve this income? What is it going to cost you to run your business? Working out how much you spend each month may be relatively easy if you are diligent with your household finances, or it may come as a shock if you are rather *laissez faire* with your money. Activity 4.1 may help with this.

✎ ACTIVITY 4.1: Your personal outgoings

Make a list of *everything* you spend in one month, probably, but not exclusively, including the following:

Mortgage/rent/council tax for your home	
Electricity, gas, water, other utilities	
Telephones (landline and mobile), broadband	
Building and contents insurance	
Home repairs and scheduled improvements	
Groceries and household shopping	
Daily living expenses, e.g., meals and parking at work	
Car expenses – fuel, repairs, insurance, tyres	
Clothing, hairdressing, beauty treatments, personal items	
Gym membership, private health insurance, other regular expenses	
Children – e.g., school fees, trips, sports and leisure activities	
Pets – food, insurance, veterinary bills	
Entertainment and holidays	
Other essential expenses	
Other non-essential expenses	

Costs of setting up your business

You will have planned what you want to offer and how you intend to provide your services (from your activities in Chapters 1 and 2), and it is now time to start spending money on making your plans a reality. You must work out *all* the costs involved in starting up your private practice – every last one. Do not under-estimate what you will need to spend in order to establish yourself and your client base to provide you with an acceptable income. Importantly, you need to identify what you should spend your limited start-up budget on and what *not* to spend it on.

Identify which aspects of the start-up process you are unable to do well yourself – and be prepared to pay for them. It is often said that one 'must speculate to accumulate', and this is certainly true of business. Trying to do everything yourself is counter-productive – it will take more time in the long run to learn how to complete some tasks than paying an expert to do this for you, for example, setting up your website or designing your logo. This could cost you more because you will be using your own time, which may be better spent elsewhere. You also risk poorly presented elements that will look unprofessional. Further, you may jeopardise your practice from the outset if you have, unknowingly, contravened some aspect of the law.

There will be some start-up costs that are common to most fledgling businesses and you may think of others that relate to the specific services you wish to offer. Count *everything*, from the largest expenditure to the most trivial.

Training and education

Here you can include any courses you have done since your initial qualification (continuing professional development (CPD)) that directly relate to your intended business services. This should include any courses you have done recently prior to making the decision to work for yourself – but you need to be able to show evidence of payment for these courses, even if only via your credit card statement if you have not kept the receipts. Courses you attend will depend on the services you want to provide but may include learning how to perform tongue-tie division, paying for yourself to attend an 'Examination of the New-born' course or complementary therapy training. You are not permitted to set the costs of your primary qualification against your tax matters – for example, university tuition fees for midwifery or your basic doula training costs – because these qualifications are fundamental to being able to offer your intended private services. Similarly, you are unable to claim for those courses that have been funded by your employer.

You should also account for any necessary courses preparing you to set up in business as well as those that are professionally relevant. For example, you may need to develop your computer skills to enable you to use specific software or programs. It is worth searching for short courses that may be offered at low cost or even free of charge by your local council, tax office, business organisation, further education department or local university. If you intend to manage your own accounts, you may decide to take a bookkeeping course to learn how to record your finances in a suitable manner for your accountant. Whilst there are many sources of help available online, it can be useful to attend some of these courses, not only for the opportunity to discuss issues in depth, but also as a means of meeting other local people starting up in business. Joining a networking group is an ideal way of finding local businesses to help you (see Chapter 5).

Research and related expenses

This may involve market research to find out what services expectant and new parents may need and for which they are prepared to pay, research on the possible competition you may have and the fees they charge, searching for the professional services you may require to ensure that you can work with them and to gauge what they will cost, or academic research for clinical evidence to support any claims you make for your services (particularly important for your marketing literature and website; see Chapter 5). Much of this can be done online, but some aspects may require some 'legwork' – for example, visiting local general practitioners (GPs) to find out if they would publicise your services, or even perhaps going for a treatment with a practitioner who provides services similar to those you intend to offer, such as a massage for relaxation (yes, enjoy it, but claim it as a legitimate business expense!). 'Research' could also include subscriptions to journals or professional database websites so that you have ready access to contemporary evidence to support your treatments.

Insurance and financial advice

This must, of course, include personal professional indemnity insurance but may also require a change of your vehicle insurance if you intend to use your own car and/or your home buildings, and contents insurance if you wish to work from home. You may also need public liability and other more specific cover depending on your personal circumstances. See Chapter 3 for more on insurance matters.

Depending on your age and personal circumstances, it is wise to explore your pension options or other investments if you are no longer employed. You may find an independent financial advisor (IFA) who offers a complimentary half-hour initial consultation to help you with this[1] – IFAs are independent of any specific business selling financial services and are able to advise and sell products from any provider right across the market, ensuring that they are tailored to your personal circumstances.

You should also invest in a will or seek help to revise an existing one. Will writing, especially if you are a director of a limited company or part of a formal partnership agreement, is an essential component of business succession planning, and not having one can complicate tax issues and probate in the event of your death. You should try to find a will writer who specialises in complex cases including advising people in business and who can advise you on minimising the potential tax liability related to your business that your heirs may face after your death. It is important to have in place an emergency plan if you die or are incapacitated to such an extent that you are no longer able to run your business. A formal process for selecting a successor to

1   To find an IFA, see www.independent-financial-advisor-uk.com and for more information on pensions for the self-employed, see www.moneyadviceservice. org.uk/en/articles/pensions-for-the-self-employed

your business, if appropriate, will also help to deal with your estate. Consult your solicitor who may refer you to a colleague who specialises in will writing, or find an independent will writer in your area.[2]

Legalities

You may need to pay for a Disclosure and Barring Service (DBS) check (formerly Criminal Records Bureau, CRB).[3,4] You will also need to register with Companies House if you are establishing a limited company.[5] If you intend to play music via any media during your relaxation sessions or antenatal classes you must have a music licence.[6] See Chapter 3 for more on the legal aspects of setting up in business.

Loans to start your business

You may decide to use some of your own savings to get started, but this should be clearly noted in your accounts. If you set up a limited company this is considered to be a director's loan (you will be the company director), and you should eventually be able to repay yourself for the monies loaned to the business. Otherwise, you may apply for a loan from your bank or building society – many schemes for new business owners are offered at a low interest rate so they can be cost-effective. Other sources of financial support for start-up businesses include Funding Circle,[7] or you could investigate whether it is possible to obtain a government grant.[8]

2   www.willwriters.com

3   www.gov.uk/request-copy-criminal-record

4   For information on registration with the Information Commissioner's Office (ICO) for data protection (General Data Protection Registration, GDPR), see https://ico.org.uk/for-organisations/guide-to-the-general-data-protection-regulation-gdpr

5   www.gov.uk/government/organisations/companies-house

6   www.gov.uk/licences-to-play-background-music

7   www.fundingcircle.com/uk/businesses

8   http://smallbusiness.co.uk/financing/government-grants or the Prince's Trust if you are under 30 years of age, www.princes-trust.org.uk/help-for-young-people/support-starting-business

In order to obtain funding, you will need to produce a clear business plan including a detailed financial forecast (see below). It is better to ask for help with this at the start to ensure a successful application rather than to try to do it yourself and have your application rejected – your bank may have local business advisors to help you.

I was very fortunate when I set up Expectancy that I did not need to apply for a bank loan. My brother and I had received a legacy and were able to fund the start-up without needing a bank loan. We put £45,000 into the business but were able to repay ourselves within the first two years of trading; £45,000 may seem like a huge amount of money – but be warned – it does not actually go very far once you start spending. I am proud to say that I have never had to ask for a bank loan, a factor that works favourably with the bank because I owe them nothing. Very occasionally I have had to put in a few extra thousand pounds as an additional, temporary director's loan when times were lean, but I have always been able to reclaim my personal money within a relatively short period of time.

Office equipment and furniture

If you intend to work from home your consulting room must have a coordinated professional appearance. You may need to purchase a new or bigger desk and comfortable chair plus a bookcase and filing cabinet. Perhaps there is a need for redecoration and new carpeting, and you may wish to purchase some suitable pictures or posters and notice boards to brighten the room and to enable you to work comfortably and professionally. You may require suitable lighting that can be dimmed for relaxation sessions or brightened for clinical procedures as appropriate. It is easy to think that these are not legitimate business expenses because they are part of your own home, but they are very necessary costs to get you started. If you rent a space in a designated clinic, or if you choose to open your own clinic, you may also need to pay for professional signage.

Website

Having a professional website developed and maintained is crucial in this day and age. Unless you have a friend or family member who is a web designer, this is an expense worth paying. Do not attempt to design your own website or do it cheaply because this will be obvious to potential visitors to your site and may give an impression that could be detrimental to your business. You may also decide to pay for the services of a graphic designer to help with the website (see Chapter 5 on websites).

Technology

You will need a mobile telephone specifically for your business and an answering machine for your landline if you do not already have one. Also consider whether you need to upgrade your desktop computer or purchase a tablet computer for use if you visit women in their own homes. You will need a printer and a range of relevant software packages, including accountancy systems, as well as intensive virus protection if you intend to keep client details on your computer. You should arrange for access to the Cloud to store your essential documents – a small amount of space is often free. If you already have access to Cloud computing you may need to pay for additional space.

Marketing

This will include printed advertising literature if you decide to use it, information leaflets for expectant parents, your personal business cards, client appointment cards and record sheets (see Chapter 5).

Professional items

If you are intending to provide physical treatments or examinations, you may need to include the purchase of a massage couch or reflexology chair, as well as aromatherapy and massage oils, towels in a coordinated colour and paper couch rolls to cover the couches.

Teaching models such as a doll and pelvis will be needed if you are going to offer antenatal classes, as well as other items such as posters. If you are working peripatetically you will need sanitising gel or hand wipes, kept in a suitably professional-looking carrying bag or case for transport of equipment between appointments. You should also carry a first aid kit. Depending on the services you offer, you may decide to purchase a sphygmomanometer and fetal Sonicaid if appropriate. You may wish to wear specialist clothing or uniform – and a name badge is essential. You will need a professional diary for your appointments – one that is separate from both your personal and your work diary if you are still working part time in the NHS. You may want to play music so you need to account for the cost of purchasing suitable music and a music licence if it is not royalty-free, as well as a machine on which you can play it (you may prefer to play it from your computer or mobile telephone, but will still need a licence).

If you have not already done so, start saving *every single receipt* for all items, services or other costs incurred in developing and setting up your business. Most of these items can be offset against tax in the first couple of years of trading, so it is really important to take account of even the most trivial expenditure – for example, every coffee you buy when meeting colleagues or attending networking events, every minor parking expense, every notepad or pen you use for your fledgling business. It all adds up in the end – one meeting a week for 40 weeks a year, at which you buy a coffee and two hours' parking, could be around £5 a week or over £200 a year.

Activity 4.2 may help you to think about your possible outgoings at the start of the business. Identify *all* the costs involved in starting up your practice. Some suggestions are given but there may be other costs not detailed below, according to the types of services you wish to offer. *Do not under-estimate how much you will spend!*

✎ ACTIVITY 4.2: Costs incurred in setting up your business

Item	Cost (£)
Initial training and education if appropriate (initial training may not be tax-deductible)	
Training to prepare you to start your business	
Research and related expenses	
Insurance	
Legalities	
Licences	
Professional services – accountant, solicitor	
Loans to start your business	
Cost of renting a room or making changes to your house to work from home	
Office equipment and furniture	
Website and graphic designer	
Technology – equipment, software, etc.	
Marketing – literature, advertising, business cards, etc.	
Professional items and equipment	
Other	

Costs of running your business on a day-to-day basis

Once you have set up your business, there will be regular ongoing costs involved in maintaining it. It is vital to budget accordingly, otherwise you may not have enough in your account to pay for essential services that must be paid regularly, such as website hosting or broadband fees. Obviously, the more clients you have, the most costs you will have, but these do not increase exponentially and eventually your income should be greater than your expenditure (otherwise your business will fail!).

Premises

If you decide to rent a room in a clinic or even to purchase a building from which to set up your own clinic, you must account for the rental and/or mortgage payments. Furthermore, if you are opening your own clinic it is likely that there will be start-up costs incurred in making the premises accessible for people with disabilities and ensuring adequate fire escapes. Depending on the services you provide, there may be other requirements such as fire-retardant paint on the walls, or issues to address that enable you to comply with Care Quality Commission (CQC) criteria if appropriate.

Professional services

These will include accountancy and possibly also bookkeeping services, and you may occasionally need the services of a solicitor. You should develop contacts who can maintain and revise your website and a graphic designer for updating photographs, logos and other visual material. Many of these services can be paid for in monthly instalments, making it easier to manage. Membership of business organisations such as the Federation of Small Businesses often entitles you to discounted fees for some of these services.

Technology

Although you will have accounted for the purchase of your mobile telephone, computer, printer and software, you must ensure that it is all kept up-to-date and working efficiently, including comprehensive, up-to-date virus protection, and you may pay an IT specialist to analyse your website visitor numbers and profiles. You could have regular fees to pay for the maintenance of specialist equipment if you have decided to rent this. Depending on how you intend to take payment from your clients you may also need to pay for machines that enable you to take debit or credit card payments, or specialist software to help you manage your client appointments.

Legalities

If you become a limited company you will need to pay an annual registration to Companies House; this is not very much, but still needs to be costed. You may need to pay for annual registration and a permit to provide specialist services from your own home, such as massage or acupuncture. If you have dedicated business premises, you will have business rates to pay. Registration with the Information Commissioner's Office (ICO) for data protection will also need to be factored in to your outgoings.

Marketing and advertising

As your business progresses you will need to budget for additional business cards, reprinting of paperwork such as client information leaflets, clinical record sheets, appointment cards and other administrative items. Money can, however, be saved here by having digital formats for most of these items – but you may then have to reconsider data protection issues.

Insurance

You will certainly need professional indemnity insurance (possibly more than one type) as it is illegal to practise without it, public liability and other insurance, most of which are paid annually (see Chapter 3).

You should also account for your personal *National Insurance contributions* if this is your only source of income (it will be taken out at source if you are in other paid employment, but you will still need to complete an online self-assessment tax return each year). If you earn enough to pay Income Tax, make sure you keep enough in your account to be able to pay this. Directors of limited companies generally have their personal tax returns completed by the accountant who deals with their company accounts, so discuss your National Insurance contributions with them.

Travel

You must record all the fuel you have used in the course of your day-to-day business activities, as well as parking, tolls and if relevant, public transport. You are not permitted to claim for car maintenance and servicing or items such as new tyres, nor for your car tax and insurance. You may claim mileage (£0.45 per mile for the first 10,000 miles and then at £0.25 per mile within any given tax year, at the time of writing[9]). You are strongly advised not to change your car classification from a personal to a company car, which has several tax disadvantages, unless your company is extremely large or you are providing services for which you require a specifically modified vehicle in order to run your business. Remember to claim for *all mileage* related to your business including visits to professionals such as your solicitor or graphic designer and to the bank, even if you are then going on to somewhere else for a personal reason, such as collecting the children from school.

Office supplies

Keep a record of all the ink cartridges, paper, pens, marker pens, notepads, whiteboards, year planners and other items you may need on a regular basis.

---

9   Check this at www.gov.uk/government/publications/rates-and-allowances-travel-mileage-and-fuel-allowances/travel-mileage-and-fuel-rates-and-allowances

Continuing professional development

You may need to undertake further training relevant to your clinical services as well as business training. Any courses, conferences or study days that you attend to enable you to revalidate with the Nursing and Midwifery Council (NMC) can now be offset against tax if you are offering services which require you to have current midwifery registration.

Professional memberships and subscriptions

You are entitled to claim back any tax on payments made for NMC registration, Royal College of Midwives (RMC) membership, Doula UK registration (or other), Federation of Small Businesses or other organisations. These are all directly relevant to your new practice – just because you paid for them yourself whilst you were employed elsewhere should not deter you from claiming them as legitimate business expenses. If you belong to a professional register for your particular services, for example, a register of lactation consultants or baby massage teachers or a specific complementary therapy organisation, you should also include this in your budget. Even if you previously paid for your own subscriptions to your preferred professional journals (midwifery/doula/medical), these now become essential business expenses. It is vital to remain up-to-date with what is happening in your professional field so that you can provide contemporary, evidence-based services, thus you can completely justify putting these costs on to your business expenditure. You should also include here any business journals to which you subscribe, any professional databases you may need to access for research papers and charges incurred for your business bank account that can be set against tax.

Networking

Membership of any groups that offer the opportunity to meet other business owners, other midwives or doulas from your own professional group, as well as groups where you may meet prospective clients, can be very productive (see Chapter 5 for more on networking).

And remember – just because you may enjoy attending these meetings does not mean you have to fund them yourself!

Clothing allowance

Expenses incurred for clothing that have a company logo and are generally used solely for the business can be claimed against tax.

Regular monthly costs

Include any costs to operate your business on a day-to-day basis, including energy costs (lighting, heating, water, electricity or gas), telephones (landline and mobile), broadband and internet access, time taken for meetings, refreshments for the office and for business meetings. If you work from home, some of these costs will be retrieved through your self-assessment tax return since you are permitted to claim a certain amount towards the use of your home as an office. This is usually a proportion of your household bills including electricity, gas, council tax and mortgage payments, but your accountant will advise you on this.

Expenses previously accounted for when you were employed

Include in your budgeting and pricing an allowance for holidays, sickness or injury, maternity or paternity leave, payments into a pension, jury service and unanticipated events such as major car or computer breakdown. Not only will you not be paid during any periods that you do not work, you may also need to pay a colleague to cover for you, and time away from your business can be costly.

Staff or freelance support

It is unlikely, at least in the beginning, that you will be considering employing staff, but you may choose to pay other people to support you. For example, you may decide to have a cleaner to ensure that your consulting room and any areas traversed by clients (such as your hallway and bathroom) are clean and tidy – this is a legitimate business expense. Many people in business also pay for the services of a virtual assistant to manage their diaries, take referrals and requests for appointments from potential clients and deal with invoicing and receipts.

If you decide to employ staff, you are legally required to pay at least the minimum wage and the employer's contribution to National Insurance and to have in place a pension plan for each employee if you have more than five. If your employee is sick, pregnant or injured at work you will have contributions to pay towards any benefits to which they may be entitled, not all of which is repaid by the government. You need employers' insurance and will also undoubtedly require the services of a solicitor.

Any other extraneous expenses

Just to reiterate…items purchased to set up and maintain the business can be claimed against your annual tax return, so retain *all* receipts – even the smallest! You may also be able to save money for your personal activities by combining them with your business ones. A good example here is to combine personal trips with travelling around for work – so if you need to go to the supermarket, do it on your way home from seeing clients, when the mileage expenditure can be claimed against your company expenses.

When you first start building your business you may not yet know what your monthly outgoings are likely to be, so you may prefer to leave Activity 4.3 until later. However, whenever you identify a new cost you can add it to the list and save it for future reference and budgeting. Here you can list all the costs you will have on a regular monthly, quarterly or annual basis in relation to keeping your business afloat. Again, as with the set-up costs, do not under-estimate what you will spend on your business. You should also allow a little extra to budget for opportunities that come along unexpectedly, such as having a stand or stall at an expectant parents' exhibition.

🔖 ACTIVITY 4.3: Ongoing costs of maintaining and running your practice

Premises	
Professional services	
Technology	
Legalities	
Marketing and advertising	
Insurance	
Travel	
Office supplies	
Continuing professional development	
Professional memberships and subscriptions	
Networking	
Clothing allowance	
Expenses previously accounted for in your employment	
Staff or freelance support	
Monthly costs	
Any other extraneous expenses	

Bank accounts

Although it is not a legal requirement for a sole trader to have a business bank account, it is wise to open a new account for the income and expenditure associated with your practice. Initially, the account can be opened in your own name but should be kept entirely for business purposes. Later, whilst there are additional charges involved in having a business bank account, you may save money on your accountancy fees because it will be easier for your accountant to analyse the income and outgoings than if everything is muddled in with your personal money.

You may be able to find a bank that offers free banking for the first year of your business and perhaps one that also pays interest on the account. If, later, you need to apply for finance from the bank, having a business account makes things easier, especially if you set up a partnership and require other signatories on the account. Having a business account also means that you are allocated a business manager who can provide advice and information on other aspects of running your business. Charges incurred for your business bank account are part of your business expenses.

If you set up as a limited company, you are legally required to have a company bank account, but look around for the best deals that may offer you some free banking at the start. Membership of certain business organisations, such as the Federation of Small Businesses, may be able to offer special deals so long as you continue your membership. Make sure that your bank account permits instant access, although if you can find an account that also pays you interest, so much the better. In this case you may have both an instant access current account and a reserve (savings) account. If you need to request a start-up bank loan you will need to draw up a business plan (see Chapter 2). Where groups of colleagues intend to work together, you may need to open a joint account with several signatories – this will normally be under the limited company arrangement in any case.

Setting your prices

Deciding on how much you are going to charge – and physically taking the money from clients – are two of the most difficult aspects of running your own business for those of us who have worked in the caring professions and particularly in an NHS culture in which services are free at the point of access. *Do not* be altruistic. This is your business, and clients *expect* to pay fees in keeping with the current market price for services offered. You may have a moral conflict with the word 'profit', but if your business is going to be successful you must, to use the modern idiom, 'get over it'. Profit provides your earnings and if you cannot resolve any internal conflicts, then running your own business may not be for you.

Think about your current salary and what you are being paid to do. If you have worked for the NHS the inherent culture discourages staff from valuing the services they provide, yet you *are* being paid for your expertise and experience. To put this in the context of starting your business, you need to look at what people choose to pay for, how much they are prepared to pay and what they identify as their priorities and also as value for money. Some people think nothing of paying £250 for a pair of trousers or £100 for a hair or beauty appointment; others choose to spend their money on long-haul overseas holidays or a sports car.

It is all very individual but pregnancy and early parenthood is often a time when families are prepared to spend more on preparing for the arrival of their baby and less, perhaps, on going out. Independent midwives will tell you that some women who initially appear, outwardly, to have much less disposable income than others will choose to pay for their services because that is what they see as a priority in their lives at that time (personal communications with independent midwives). Of course, your market is going to be one in which your clients can afford to pay you, unless you set up as a social enterprise scheme (see Chapter 2). You may decide that you want to offer some discounted fees for those in need who are unable to pay your fees – but in this case you should consider increasing your prices for everyone else to part-cover your losses from free or heavily discounted services.

If, from the first interaction with potential clients, you are clear about the fees you charge, this gives them the option not to use your services if they feel it is more than they can afford. When they telephone for an appointment, tell them how much it will be and if there are any other potential costs, for example, oil blends, wristbands for nausea or 'hypnobirthing' CDs. However, it may depend on what you are offering – parents may prefer to pay £200 for a practitioner to perform tongue-tie division on their three-day-old baby rather than waiting six weeks for an NHS appointment, or £60 per appointment for a course of acupuncture treatment for pelvic girdle pain instead of joining the long queue for an NHS physiotherapy appointment. Doulas, in particular, are increasingly in demand to assist families before, during and after the birth, and some charge up to £4000 for their services. I know of one doula who recently informed me that she had paid an annual tax bill to HMRC in excess of £10,000, meaning that she was earning at least £50,000 a year.

It is also important to try to work out how many clients you need to see in order that your business can break even and how much business you need to make a profit. Your break-even point is the point at which your total income equals your total expenses for any given period. At this point there is no profit or loss – in other words, you 'break even'. Knowing your break-even point will help you when setting your prices and budgets for the year and, if appropriate, when preparing a business plan. It can help you to identify which aspects of your practice are profitable, how many clients you need to see in order to make a profit, and the point at which you will start to make a loss if business is poor.

When pricing your services, you should take into consideration that fees need to reflect both your outgoings and the minimum income on which you need to live, whilst offering a service that is value for money for the client. Prices need, at the very least, to take account of your start-up costs and maintenance fees (usually spread over a two- or three-year period), your equipment and general running costs *and* your time. When calculating how much your time is worth, try not to think what you believe people will pay, but consider what they will be getting.

It is paramount to the success of your business to understand and appreciate what your services are worth – and try never to compete on price. You are a highly trained professional, possibly with several years' experience in your particular field, and it is that for which your clients choose to pay. You have already dedicated much time and money to your initial and subsequent training and to setting up your business. You are providing services that your prospective clients want, often services that are not readily available on the NHS. You are giving them time and the opportunity to talk, to ask you questions and to receive information and advice. You must remember to include in your calculations the time you spend in travelling to and between appointments, the days when you are not earning, such as when you are attending a conference or going to networking events, as well as your holidays and any possible sickness. *Do not under-estimate this.*

You should also account for the occasional incident when a client fails to pay you (see below). Change your mind-set and come to terms with the commercial world beyond the protected environment of state-funded employment. In other words, do not under-sell or under-value yourself! It is your livelihood, and not charging enough may make the difference between success and failure.

The fees you decide to charge may, of course, vary according to the geographical area in which you live and work and the services you are providing. Inner-city prices, especially in London and other large conurbations, will be considerably more than in rural areas. Conversely, increased competition in large cities may mean that other practitioners charge lower prices, but this is usually offset by increased demand. These factors may impact on the way you work, for example, whether you have a static base for your clients to come to you, or whether you choose to be peripatetic. If you provide basic relaxation massage treatments for pregnancy, it would not be wise to price yourself excessively above other antenatal massage therapists in your area. However, if you are offering specialist services – such as natural treatments for post-dates pregnancy or moxibustion for breech presentation – then you have what is called a 'unique selling point' or USP. This means that there are fewer practitioners, or none at all, offering these services, and women will come to you because they have a specific need. Similarly, if your doula services include some little 'extras' that set you aside from other colleagues, you will be able to advertise your more specialist services – and charge more than the competition.

Also, whilst we would not want women to experience severe problems, they can sometimes be so desperate to get help that they may be prepared to travel long distances for your services. I once had a client with excessive nausea and vomiting (not diagnosed as hyperemesis gravidarum) who set off from Manchester to London to see me. Unfortunately, she only reached as far as Oxfordshire because she felt so unwell that she was admitted to the local hospital, but it was a mark of the severity of her symptoms that she chose to attempt the journey.

You may decide to charge by the hour or per treatment. It is wise to charge more for services not generally available in your area or for which there is a long waiting list with the NHS. In London an hour's treatment could be around £60, but in other areas it may more realistically be £40–£50 per hour. However, you would need to charge more for a shorter session – so a 30-minute appointment might be priced at £25–£35 rather than £20–£30. The first appointment will usually take longer because you need to take a comprehensive history from the woman, so this should be priced accordingly. Classes and group sessions will usually be less per person per hour but *always* charge for a full course of classes rather than on a sessional basis – if someone is unable to attend one of the sessions, you will already have been paid. You should also make a small charge for any accompanying person – and again, include this in the overall cost of the course of classes.

If your practice involves travelling to women's own homes, you should include mileage in your calculations. You could decide on a radius of, say, 15 miles from your base and then charge an extra £1 per mile for anyone requesting your services who lives outside this boundary. I once had a client who lived on the Surrey/Hampshire border who booked a course of treatment for severe nausea and vomiting; I drove from South London on three occasions to treat her, a round trip of some 120 miles. In this case I charged her mileage in addition to the normal consultation fees and she was happy to pay this. I have even had a woman from France who wanted me to travel to her near Calais but sadly she miscarried before I could manage to see her.

You also need to account for the time you spend in travelling between appointments, not just the cost of fuel. This must be factored into your diary – and will probably mean that the number of clients you see in a day will be limited unless you live and work in a very urbanised area (although traffic problems must also be considered). Many years ago, when I was first starting to work privately, I had a client who requested an appointment for nausea and vomiting and who lived approximately 40 minutes' drive away from my home. I gave her a price of just £60, which seemed reasonable to me and to which she agreed. Unfortunately, the motorway route to her area was closed due to an accident, necessitating a detour through various villages. However, this was a Saturday in December and it seemed that all the villages were having their Christmas fayres; consequently, the minor roads were also blocked. It took me three-and-a-half hours to reach the client, I spent an hour-and-a-half with her and then drove home, almost another hour. One appointment, for which I had charged £60, had taken me six hours – equating to £10 per hour! This did not even cover the cost of the fuel, paperwork, insurance and equipment, let alone my training, expertise and time. Needless to say, I increased my prices considerably after that – and women were still prepared to pay the fees.

Sometimes you will find that charging a little more can be very productive – and this is not meant to be avaricious. Think about the way in which you might consider the purchase of a new washing machine – you probably compare prices on several models but also examine quality, features, longevity and brand. When pared down to about three different products, most people tend to opt for the middle-priced product, a few will opt for the more expensive one, but fewer will buy the cheapest model unless cost is the primary – perhaps the only – deciding factor. People seem to feel that they are getting more when they pay more, and if you feel you can offer value for money, then it is worth a trial, if nothing else. It is also very difficult if you start your practice with low prices then decide you need to increase them; plus people may not trust you if you set your prices below the current market price for similar services. Start with a realistic price and test the market – you might be pleasantly surprised.

It is normal to consider a price increase in line with inflation at the beginning of each trading year. This point may be the start of the calendar year or the financial year (6 April), or the date on which your practice commenced, especially if you decide to form a limited company or partnership. I know of a doula who increases her prices after every tenth client: she sees about 15 a year, so the price increase is approximately every eight to nine months, yet she continues to grow her business. It is interesting to note, however, that doulas generally have a far more realistic approach to charging for their services because they are trained to work in private practice. It is normally the midwives who have never had to deal with money in the NHS who have more difficulty in this area. Even those involved in setting budgets often distance the concept of money from its relationship to clients. It can be difficult for NHS employees to appreciate the immense costs involved in running a business, and it may not be until you start up yourself that you will understand just how fine a balance it can be between success and failure.

You might be inclined to offer discounts if a woman books several treatments together (e.g., six sessions for the price of five), but try to avoid doing this. You may believe that it brings clients flocking to your door, but you will still have the costs of the extra sessions to absorb into your charges. Some clients may ask if they can pay in instalments and this can be good practice because they are then more likely to book with you. However, you should have in place a formal written agreement so that they understand that they are committed to paying the full amount, irrespective of whether they complete the course of treatment or classes. Perhaps you could offer alternatives – for example, a woman who books a course of six antenatal treatments for backache who then goes into labour before the course is completed could be offered relaxation treatments in the postnatal period as a replacement for the missed sessions.

There are just three factors that affect how much you will earn: the number of customers, your expenses and your prices. To achieve an increase in your income you must increase the number of clients (customers), increase your prices (income) or reduce your expenses (outgoings). In order to set your prices appropriately you need to take into account all the issues discussed above, cost out your expenses and then decide on a fee that the local market will pay. Activities 4.4 and 4.5 are designed to help you with this.

✎ ACTIVITY 4.4: Calculating your workload

1. From your list of the services you wish to provide (refer back to Chapter 1 if necessary), calculate the amount of time required for each type of consultation, then average this between the different types of services you will offer.

2. Depending on whether you are going to be static (in your own home or based in a clinic setting) or peripatetic (visiting women in their homes), you now need to consider how many hours you could feasibly work in a single day. There may be more time if you work in a clinic rather than accounting for travel time between home visits, but you must also think about your own energy levels and how this may affect your ability to see more clients.

3. Now decide how many days a week you wish to work in your practice and how many weeks of the year. You may prefer not to work in school holidays, or you may want to take a three-day weekend every week. You should now have the total number of hours to be worked in a year.

4. Now divide the total number of hours per year (as in (2) and (3)) by the average amount of time required for your range of services (as in (1)) to give you the total number of client sessions you should be able to see in a year.

Example:

- Average duration of appointments – 1.5 hours (no. 1)

- Maximum number of hours per year – 4 per day x 4 days per week x 45 weeks of the year = 720 (nos 2 and 3)

- 720 hours divided by 1.5 hours per average appointment = 480 clients per year (no. 4)

5. From Activities 4.2 and 4.3, calculate the approximate costs you will incur in the first two years of your business. Your initial start-up costs should be spread across both years, so if you spend £10,000 to set up your business, that would be £5000 per year, plus the annual costs of running your business on a day-to-day basis.

6. Now, assuming you are working as a sole trader, add an extra 20 per cent on any amount in excess of the personal allowance of £11,000 (tax year 2017–18) to cover Income Tax.

7. Divide the annual costs in (5) by the total number of clients you could see in a year (from no. 4). This gives you the average price you need to charge for your consultations in order to break even.

8. Now add on a reasonable percentage to enable you to make a profit – for example, a 25 per cent increase in the average price of each consultation.

   Example over the first two years of trading:

   – Start-up costs £10,000 over two years = £5000 per year

   – Annual ongoing costs £1000 per month x 12 = £12,000

   – Ongoing costs £12,000 plus start-up costs = £17,000 per year

- Plus 20% Income Tax on £6000 = £1200 per year = £18,200

- £18,200 divided by 480 clients per year = £38 average consultation cost

- Plus 25% to £47.50 per treatment to provide a profit

If you feel that this is too much to expect someone to pay for your services, you must either increase the number of women you see, reduce the appointment time, or take less profit.

Taking payments

You now need to decide how you will require your clients to pay you. When a prospective client contacts you, make clear the fees she will be expected to pay and how you will accept payment. It can feel embarrassing to ask a woman face-to-face to pay you for the services, particularly if you accept cash payments (although taking payment in cash is not recommended as it can be difficult to monitor it). Bank transfers paid in advance of the appointment or series of consultations may be a good way to guarantee payment and ensures a commitment of the woman to attend, unless she is unwell. If you develop into a large practice and choose to use a software package for managing your appointments, this may include a system whereby pre-payment is required to confirm the appointment. Certain mobile telephone applications can also enable you to take payments at the point of contact with clients, such as iZettle or smartTrade. If you are prepared to accept payment by credit or debit card, you could consider PayPal or a similar system, although there will be a small fee to be paid for this service. If you decide to take credit or debit card payments at the point of contact, there is a fee to be paid both for rental of the equipment and for each transaction, equivalent to approximately 4 per cent of the transaction cost. Membership of some business organisations such as the Federation of Small Businesses may include benefits such as reduced fees for taking card payments. Any fees that you are required to pay for these services should either be factored in across all fees charged or added to the invoice as a convenience charge for clients wishing to use this method of payment.

Legally, the client must pay you within 30 days of the service being provided, and you are entitled to charge a late payment penalty, but this should be made clear on your invoice or contract. Pregnant women are notoriously forgetful, so it is better to implement a system that requires them to pay in advance or at the start or end of the appointment rather than risk not being paid at all. Your written cancellation policy should also include your expectations if a woman cancels or forgets her appointment, gives birth or experiences an emergency that means she cannot attend (see Chapter 3 for more on contracts with clients).

Invoices and receipts

An invoice is a statement detailing what monies will be required; a receipt acknowledges that payment has been made. It can be easier to present clients with an invoice for payment say, within seven days, than asking for direct payment. It is good practice to offer a receipt to confirm that payment has been made. This system of invoices and receipts also helps your bookkeeping system and makes it easier to track back, against your diary, to ensure that everyone has paid and that you have a complete record of monies due. This can also mean that the money is paid by direct bank transfer, obviating the need to ask for money in person – you can just present the client with the invoice.

Any written request for payment must state clearly that it is an invoice and there must be a unique, sequential identification number. You must also include your company name, registered address and contact information (email and telephone), as well as the name and address of the customer you are invoicing. There must be a clear description of the service you are providing, with the date the services are due to be provided (the supply date) and the date of the invoice issue. You must state the amount being charged, together with any Value Added Tax (VAT), if applicable (see below). If there are several elements to the service or product provision, these must be itemised separately and a total amount due identified on the invoice.

If you are a sole trader, you must also include your own name and the business name, together with an address where any legal documents can be delivered to you if you are using a business name. If you have a limited company, the full name, as it appears on the certificate of incorporation from Companies House, must be included. If you decide to add the names of the company directors on your invoices (not essential), you must include the names of all directors, even those who are not actively involved in the day-to-day business of the company. If you are registered for VAT you must use specific VAT invoices with your VAT number on them). If, however, you are providing services to individuals who are not VAT-registered, you do not need to provide a full VAT invoice, although it is usually easier to do so.

Receipts provide a record that payment has been received and act as the client's proof of purchase. It is useful to issue both an invoice and a receipt to the client, and to keep copies of these for your records. Receipts should show the date (and time) of the service provision, the type and number of services or products purchased, the name and location of the business, any VAT charged and the method of payment. If appropriate, you may also need to include a returns policy (for any products you may sell). The receipt may be in either hard copy (paper format) or sent via email, the latter of course being cheaper, but ensure that you keep a record that it has been sent/received/read.

Dealing with Her Majesty's Revenue & Customs

You will need to maintain *diligently* any records pertaining to your income and outgoings, for HMRC. If you are a sole trader, it is not essential to use the services of an accountant or a bookkeeper, especially if this is not your sole source of income. However, you will need to speak to your tax office (usually Glasgow for current NHS employees) and ask them to register you for self-assessment. You will need to complete an online self-assessment return annually and submit it by the end of October if you wish HMRC to calculate your tax for you.

As a business owner you need to submit your accounts to HMRC to ensure that you pay tax on earnings or profit. The standard tax (fiscal) year is from 6 April to 5 April of the following year. Currently, tax returns are submitted online or in hard copy annually, although your own tax year may differ from the standard April–April year, according to when you established the business and whether or not you are a sole trader or have a limited company. At the time of writing, the government has pledged to make tax digital, and there will be an obligation for all small businesses, of whatever size, to submit their accounts digitally from 2020. This process is intended to simplify the whole process of submitting tax returns, although the changeover period is currently causing major headaches for many accountants assisting micro-businesses to deal with the new system.[10]

Currently, at the end of the relevant tax year limited companies have a statutory duty to submit to HMRC their full accounts and a company tax return. There are fines of between £150 and £1500 for late submissions, although the new system should eliminate the possibility of late submissions. For limited companies, profit above a certain level incurs a payment to HMRC for Corporation Tax, which is currently 19 per cent. Sole traders do not submit a company tax return but at present file a self-assessment form online. You have until 31 January to submit your accounts, but if you wish HMRC to calculate the amount of Income Tax you owe, you must submit them by 31 October prior to this. This differentiation should disappear once digital submissions become mandatory after April 2019. Personal Income Tax is currently paid at 20 per cent on any amounts above your personal allowances, so if your business income is substantial, it

---

10 See www.gov.uk/government/uploads/system/uploads/attachment_data/file/
    413975/making-tax-easier.pdf for more information, and consult your
    accountant for further advice pertinent to your own personal and business
    circumstances.

is better to register as a limited company rather than continuing as a sole trader.

You are legally required to register for VAT if your turnover in any one year is more than £83,000 (as at 2018). Turnover is the amount of income you receive and not the profit made once expenses have been deducted. It is possible to register voluntarily for VAT before this time, which enables you to reclaim any VAT paid on goods and services for which you have paid (business expenses), but it is wise to consult your accountant on whether or not this is appropriate for your business.

You should maintain the following records for your accountant, HMRC or other official purposes:

- Record of all income from your private practice, and whether paid in cash, cheque, direct bank transfer, credit or debit card or other method.

- Your P60 form from your other sources of employment, for example, NHS – this is usually sent with your pay slip in April or May and confirms your income and your National Insurance and Income Tax payments deducted by your NHS trust in the financial year ending 5 April. *Do not* lose this form as no replacements are issued. You should keep these for at least five years.

- If you have resigned from any paid employment you will also be given a P45 form; ensure that you keep this for the next five years.

- Record of *all* outgoings for training, setting up, equipment and other items required for you to conduct your consultancy as well as mileage and other expenses paid out of your own pocket.

- Bank statements for your designated account – if you use the services of an accountant they will need to see all of these. If you use online banking facilities it is wise to print these off monthly so that you maintain a complete record as hard copy.

- P11D form of benefits (limited company directors).

Case study: Eleanor Fowler BSc

Birth and postnatal doula (www.birth-doula.co.uk), working in Oxfordshire, Buckinghamshire and Hertfordshire.

I had worked in recruitment successfully for 15 years since leaving university. In 2006 I was about to return to recruitment part time having had my third child in five years. Unfortunately, just before returning I suffered an episode of septic shock and ended up in ITU in multiple organ failure. Having nearly died and then having spent a prolonged period on life support in the high dependency unit, I needed a year to recover from the physical and mental effects. I realised there was more to life than working long hours for someone else, in a job which, although financially rewarding, was not especially fulfilling and from which I was easily replaceable.

I had considered training to be a midwife after each of my children was born, as I had wonderful birth experiences and great midwifery care. However, I repeatedly discounted this idea as the training with three small children was just not feasible. I pondered this path again but discounted it due to the similarities of working for another large organisation (the NHS), the politics, paperwork and not being able to choose when to work or with whom.

Then I read an article about doulas! I went on a preparation course through Nurturing Birth, joined Doula UK, set up my business in 2008 and have never looked back! I provide antenatal preparation and birth care, as well as postnatal doula and night nanny services. Fortunately, being a doula is not hugely expensive to set up and I left a very well-paid job, so the initial course fees were affordable.

Your greatest achievements? In nine years I have supported over 100 births, had numerous repeat clients, some of whom have genuinely become friends, have been asked to be at babies' christenings, birthdays, family gatherings and sadly funerals too. I was even asked to be one child's legal guardian if anything happened to the parents. I have supported dozens of families postnatally and learned so much from each of them. I am invited into people's homes, introduced to their cultures, beliefs and traditions, and have shared in their secrets. I have been privileged to help with single babies, multiples, parents with disabilities and babies, surrogate and adopted children and children of many different nationalities. I have been part of their lives, from celebrities to families on the edge of being homeless, and I can guarantee I have added value and will be remembered by them forever.

Your biggest mistake? My biggest mistake has been not to look after myself better and saying 'no' occasionally. Over the years I have learned I need to debrief every experience in some way, so I can let it go and not take it to the next client, whether it is taking on a family's secrets or sadness, understanding how a client may feel about her birth or postnatal journey, or trying to reassure myself that the attitude of some health professionals towards doulas is not personal. Nearly ten years on I am pretty good about letting stuff go but also asking for help or speaking out when needed. I still occasionally find myself working five days and six nights a week as I feel bad saying 'no' to a woman truly in need of support.

How has your business evolved since you first started? It hasn't changed but I know more stuff! My agreements are more formalised. My record keeping is more organised, and I am less reticent about saying 'no' occasionally. I budget every year for professional development costs. I am very fortunate to earn between £50,000 and £100,000 a year.

What is the best thing about working for yourself? Flexibility and being able to choose whom I work with and where. I can take time off for my children if I need to, I can meet friends or spend time with my husband, and I don't have to work with people I don't like!

What causes you most difficulty in running your own business? Doing my tax return! I only recently hired an accountant, which helps, but it is the one job I loathe!

What advice would you give to a midwife/doula who is just setting out in the commercial world? Network, be yourself and be totally honest and open. I do advertise, but at least 50 per cent of my clients are from referrals. When I meet a client, they see the real me. I think my recruitment experience helps, but essentially, if you are yourself and don't 'over-promise or under-deliver', you will be successful. Listen to your client, listen to colleagues, listen some more, take feedback away and reflect on it, even if you don't like it!

Any other comments? Working with people in a role like this means putting yourself aside. My opinions are rarely voiced to my clients as they are irrelevant. I often bite my tongue when saying something will make me feel better but won't help the situation.

5

Marketing Your Business

To ensure the success of your business you must take steps to tell people about your services – otherwise you will not get any clients! This is called 'marketing' and involves a process by which you tell potential clients what you have to offer in a way that entices them to investigate further and hopefully, to decide to buy from you. Marketing can be one of the most difficult aspects for a fledgling business to get right – and it does not necessarily get easier as your business grows.

Marketing includes the promotion and sale of your brand (services and goods) through various means of direct advertising. This includes your personal business cards, printed literature and information leaflets, online advertising through your website and social media and perhaps also attending exhibitions. Indirect advertising may come through writing an online blog, contributing to magazines and online resources aimed at expectant parents, speaking at meetings and classes for your potential client group and 'word of mouth' – one of the best ways of promoting yourself and your business.

Marketing that is relevant and able to reach prospective clients leads to sales. Achieving a 'sale' (i.e., successfully persuading a woman to book an appointment or buy a service from you) is dependent not only on your branding, your overt marketing strategies and the image you portray to people, but also being able to 'close the sale'. This means that you must be forward (and confident) enough to prompt enquirers into buying – it is very difficult for people to say 'no' when you ask them outright if they would like an appointment with you.

When dealing with professionals you should not, for example, merely circulate your leaflets to local general practitioner (GP) surgeries or put them in the antenatal clinic (with permission), but you should also follow them up.

The sales process requires you to:

- Seek out potential new customers (market research)

- Determine a brand for your business (branding)

- Make initial contact with potential clients (advertising)

- Communicate well what you have to offer, justifying why women should choose your services, and answering any questions on issues that may deter people from buying

- Persuade potential clients to become actual clients ('closing the sale')

- Offer an after-sales service – perhaps a telephone call to see how the client is feeling.

Market research

In order to identify if there is a market for your services and to help focus your branding and advertising appropriately you need to know what, who and where the market is, what they want and how they would like it delivered. This is called 'market research'. When you understand more about your potential and the actual market in your area you can use this information to determine how you intend to promote your services and what the market will pay (see 'Setting your prices' in Chapter 4).

Prior to commencing your market research, it is useful to have identified precisely what services you are intending to provide, by writing a mission statement – this will also be needed if you are requesting financial help from a bank or other source of funding (see Chapter 4). A mission statement is a written summary of who you are, what you offer, what benefits clients can gain from coming to you and what factors contribute to making you the 'go-to' professional for your type of services.

Market research helps you to discover:

- who your customers are – their age, occupation, lifestyle, education and the size of the market

- what they purchase in terms of maternity-related products or services and whether their needs are currently being met by existing service provision

- why they buy these services – are they looking for something not available in the NHS or are they trying to supplement or replace something in their NHS care with which they are dissatisfied?

- why they should buy from you and whether you feel able to fill a gap by offering something that is not already available or to take your share of the existing market.

The information you are seeking may be found online, in local community publications and in places where the community gathers such as church halls, local GP practices and online support groups for expectant and new parents (such as NetMums[1] and MumsNet[2]). If you work for the NHS, or with a friend who is employed by the NHS, you may also be able to get a feel for the services that women would like available – how many women ask about private antenatal classes, having a doula, accessing natural ways of getting into labour or finding sources for relaxation treatments? If you have children at school talk to parents at the school gates, visit local nurseries and maternity and babywear shops. Ask questions and talk to as many people as possible. Even just walking around some of these areas can give you some ideas about your market. Make contact with local practitioners who provide maternity-related services that may complement your own, such as baby massage instructors, pregnancy yoga teachers, and even local photographers.

It may also be useful, anonymously, to visit some of your competitors or telephone them for information about their services. Pretending to be an expectant parent or saying that you are contacting

1   www.netmums.com
2   www.mumsnet.com

them on behalf of a friend can tell you a lot about the attitude, safety, prices and availability of others who may be offering services similar to yours. Although not for market research, I once telephoned a reflexology clinic, professing to be calling on behalf of my pregnant daughter. I wanted to find out about their practices in relation to providing reflexology to initiate labour. I was horrified to discover that they would indiscriminately treat any heavily pregnant woman who walked through the door without taking any history or determining the gestation!

Analysing your potential market can be difficult, but take care not to make assumptions. Not all women will be able, or want, to pay for services not provided by the NHS. Conversely, you may be surprised at what some feel is missing from the conventional maternity services and for which they are prepared to pay. Understanding your clients' needs is fundamental to success. For example, you may know that as many as 91 per cent of women have been shown to use complementary therapies or natural remedies during pregnancy (see Tiran 2018). This may lead you to believe that women want to receive complementary therapies from their midwives. However, this may not be the case. Further searching and conversations with women might lead you to realise that what they actually want is an empathetic person who is available to talk with them, answer their questions, provide moral and informational support and consequently to reduce their fear and anxiety. Midwives' lack of time is one of the reasons why increasing numbers of women are seeking support from doulas, who generally work outside the mainstream maternity services and are available as and when women need them – and women are prepared to pay for this service (see Chapter 1 for more on the justification for private services for pregnant women).

Convincing women that they should buy from you and not someone else is about selling yourself. When you are selling your business services you are, in effect, selling yourself, even if you have staff or freelance contributors working with you. People buy people and the ways in which you interact with potential, current and past clients and their families can make all the difference to your practice. In other words, your business is a reflection of you and how you see yourself. You need to be visible, credible and have a form of personal branding (see below). It can be daunting to sell yourself, but remember that you already have experience of doing this – for example, persuading prospective employers when you attend for interviews that *you* are the person they should appoint.

Identifying a unique selling point (USP) can also be an effective marketing tool. As a lecturer, my own USP is based on my professional philosophy of adhering to safety and accountability – which is the reason why many midwives choose my courses on complementary therapies rather than those provided by other organisations (even though others may be cheaper). Focusing on the problems you can solve contributes to a USP, for example, providing services to deal with specific issues in pregnancy such as breech presentation, fear of birth or avoiding medical induction of labour. This will be more relevant to women than advertising the specific tools you may use to help women with these problems. So, when considering how to promote your services, try to put yourself in the woman's shoes – she has an issue for which she requires help and for which she generally does not know the answer.

Market research is not something you undertake only when you are starting up: once your practice is established you should periodically re-examine the market to determine whether you are still meeting the needs of your potential clients, or whether you should adapt your services and/or consider a change of direction to retain your customer base. It is important to keep up-to-date with current trends and potential changes in maternity services so that you can keep one step ahead – for example, what will be the positive and/or negative impact on your business of the incoming Personal Maternity Care Budget (PMCB)?

Ongoing market research could be in the form of surveys to your past clients or to contacts on your business social media platforms (Survey Monkey is an easy and free way to conduct a survey and obtain customer feedback[3]). You could also carry out a professional/academic search for evidence to support your services. This is not exactly *market* research but it will provide you with information on what is popularly used and the robustness of the evidence. A good source of research

---

3   www.surveymonkey.co.uk

abstracts, particularly on aspects of complementary therapies, is *CAM on PubMed*®,[4] which searches through PubMed and CINAHL to avoid the need for you to look separately at these databases.

🔖 ACTIVITY 5.1: Undertaking market research for your business

–   Consider *one* of the services you identified in Activity 2.1 (Chapter 2) as something you would like to provide in your business.

–   Now conduct an online search for the availability of this type of service in your local area. Use a variety of terms to widen your search – for example, if you are investigating 'pregnancy massage' use synonyms such as pregnancy, antenatal, fertility, expectant and massage, treatments, spa, pampering and more. (You may find some online programmes that help with this; they are usually intended for search engine optimisation (see below) – or you could use an online thesaurus.)

–   This search will help to identify services currently available and how they present themselves, highlight the ways in which the services are marketed by the competition and demonstrate whether there is a place for your own services.

Branding

You may, by now, have a name for your business and maybe even a slogan (strapline), but this is not your brand. Branding is about

---

4   https://nccih.nih.gov/research/camonpubmed

your identity. Your brand is you, your name and your logo design as well as your values and philosophy relating to the services you provide.

Having a recognisable brand helps to distinguish you from your competitors and is vital to the success of your business. It tells potential clients what they can expect from your services or products and places you in a position that is crucial to getting business (income). Branding should clearly deliver the message you wish to give out and, if done well, it helps to boost your credibility. Branding should also provide an emotional connection between your potential clients and your services, motivating them to buy and encouraging brand loyalty so that they come back for more. Of course, your branding needs to enable your customers to identify the types of services you offer, but also to help them to understand why they should use you instead of the competition.

You need to understand your potential clients and what exactly they want. Branding is about getting your potential clients to see you as the sole provider of a solution to their problem. This is why it is so important to put your marketing into terms that women can understand. Avoid professional jargon in your leaflets or on your website. For example, it is better to state that you offer 'natural induction' for women who are 'overdue' rather than using terms such as 'post-dates pregnancy'. Try not to use professional jargon at all in your marketing, including abbreviations and phrases about the service that are so much a part of our everyday professional communications. Other issues such as font styles, colours and the language used in your marketing materials, website and social media will all also affect public perception.

Developing your brand can be difficult, especially when you are first starting your business, and it is likely to evolve as your business develops and grows. If you really want to make your mark right from the start, I would advise you to seek out the services of a branding company or a graphic designer to help plan your logo, colour scheme and the graphics used to create your brand awareness. It is essential that they understand your business and what you have to offer, as well as the way that you want to work and the passions that make you tick. This can help to give you a corporate and consistent image. When I was having my website re-designed after some years in the business,

I chose a branding company to help me. I spent a wonderful afternoon with my new graphic designer making a vision board, going through magazines and other literature to identify my preferred colours, fonts, pictures and other aspects that helped her to understand what I did and the focus I wanted for the website and other marketing. Now, after many years working with both the same web and graphic designers, they know exactly what I want and are able to advise me on how to achieve it.

The questions in Activity 5.2 are designed to help you to focus on what your business is really about. Your answers will certainly help to work towards your brand, whether you choose to use professional services or to do it yourself. Your answers will also help you when writing your biography (see below).

✎ ACTIVITY 5.2: Identifying your personal brand

    — What is the fundamental *purpose* of your business?

    — *Why* did you set up your business and what are the passions that drive you?

    — How do you *present* yourself? Do you have a formal or informal approach?

– What *message* do you want to give to your clients about yourself and about your services?

– What are the core *values* that you promise to deliver to your clients?

– Why should your potential clients *believe* your promise?

– What are the short- and long-term *goals* for your business?

Designing your logo

A logo is a representation of your business that helps to build brand awareness so that people recognise the name of your company. A professional-looking logo builds trust so, even if you choose not to use professional help for your branding, asking an expert to design your logo for you is a must. I have had three different logos in the

15 years I have been in business, and it was not until I sought help from a branding company that I was truly satisfied with the logo. If it looks as if you have designed it yourself it can affect your credibility and the trust that people have in you and your services. This is far more important in today's business world than it was when I started my company in 2003 – people expect perfection, and with so much competition around in some areas, a poor logo may mean that potential clients go elsewhere.

There are several types of logo. A freestanding word or an abbreviation of the name can be used – for example, Google or IBM – or a single letter such as the 'M' for McDonald's (called a 'wordmark'). Other companies use a pictorial logo, for example, Starbucks (the two-tailed mermaid), or even an abstract – Nike's 'tick' is probably one of the most well-known brands in this latter case (these are 'brand marks'). It will depend on the name you have chosen for your business as to which type might work well for you, and is also, of course, dependent on the services you want to provide. If you have a short business name, such as eBay, you could consider a wordmark or lettermark; abstract symbols tend to be less well remembered until they have been in the public domain for some time or they are associated with one of the large public companies. Many businesses offering maternity-related services (my own included) use various representations of a mother and baby: my logo has taken the 'e' of Expectancy and depicted it as a pregnant abdomen whilst retaining the clear font of the full word.

Colour choice is vital; colour can have a psychological impact on the people who see it. Red is often considered fiery – think Red Bull energy drinks – but in advertising, it is often associated with the food industry, particularly fast food – both McDonald's and Burger King use solid red in their logos. Yellow is a 'happy' colour – so McDonald's has both red and yellow – whereas blues evoke calmness, confidence and reliability – examples here include car manufacturers such as BMW and Ford. Purple is often associated with royalty and with academia – hence the Expectancy logo is in a shade that is generally considered to be 'academic purple' because the primary business of the company is education. Green is a positive, peaceful and cool colour, and portrays relaxation; it is good for easing depression and anxiety and many therapists use it (lime, grass or sage shades) for their logos. Black and white convey power, authority and strength; pinks are feminine (or 'girly') and can have sexual connotations. Pastel shades are often associated with spring and new growth and are frequently chosen by maternity practitioners or complementary therapists. However, they can be insipid and may not be dynamic enough, especially in print, so get some expert advice on this if you are considering pastels for your logo.

Font type and size must also be considered because different fonts work for different types of business. A law firm might use a bold, straightforward font with no flourishes, whereas a sweet shop or funfair may choose a fancy, creative font that indicates fun and youth.

Activity 5.3 may help you to work out the factors that are important to you when designing your logo.

ACTIVITY 5.3: Designing your logo

- Conduct an online search for maternity-related services provided by midwives, doulas, therapists and obstetricians, as well as larger private companies.

- Look at the logo that each business has used and choose ten to fifteen different ones. There should be a mix of logos that appeal to you and those that you do not like or feel are inappropriate.

– Make a chart with each name/logo down the side and two columns along the top, labelled 'Positive' and 'Negative'.

– Now reflect on each logo and consider exactly what you feel about each one, adding your thoughts in either the 'Positive' or 'Negative' column. Think about the graphics, shapes, fonts, colours, words and sizes of each logo.

– Finally, highlight five points that have impacted on you during this exercise that have contributed to making some decisions about the kind of the logo you would like for your own business. This does not have to mean that you have actually drawn the logo by this stage, but rather, that you have come to some conclusions about the style of logo, colour and font you may prefer.

Advertising

Advertising is a component of branding. Advertising works by creating patterns of association that work emotionally to influence purchasing behaviour. The way an advertisement makes you feel can produce a long-term association with the product. Your advertising needs to portray the message that women would benefit from using your services or products rather than someone else who may be offering the same or similar services. In the 1970s, Smash was able to convince women that it was much better to use an instant mashed potato product than to spend time peeling potatoes, even though the packet product was considerably more expensive than potatoes – and it tasted awful! Clever marketing, in which strange beings from outer space found it hilarious to see humans peeling potatoes, was able to convince women, many of whom were now going out to work, to buy this time-saving product.

You do not need to spend a lot of money on advertising: it can be extremely expensive and unproductive. In the early days of my business I spent an inordinate amount of money trying to advertise across numerous journals, only to find that I was spreading myself far too thinly. It is generally held that repeated advertising in journals, with a minimum of three insertions at regular intervals, is needed for readers to recognise the logo and begin to take note of what is being offered. Nowadays I rarely pay for advertising unless there is a specific reason to do so, but with the popularity and ease of use of free social media, this is a more productive way to spread the word, as long as it is done well. Indeed, fostering good public relations, in which you develop relationships with either potential clients or professionals who can refer women to you, will bring far more in terms of boosting your professional credibility and the uniqueness of your services than paying for expensive advertising.

Advertising of any sort should be legal, fair, honest and truthful, clearly identifiable as marketing media and should not mislead the public into thinking it is something other than an advertisement. You often see advertorials in women's magazines, perhaps as an interesting article about skincare, but acting as a means of promoting a specific skin product. However, you will see in one corner of the page words such as 'for marketing purposes only' or similar, making its purpose obvious to readers.

From a professional perspective, and in line with the requirements of the Nursing and Midwifery Council (NMC), midwives are not permitted to imply in any of their advertising, in whatever form, that the possession of a qualification in midwifery results in a superior maternity-related service (NMC 2015, 21). However, it is perfectly acceptable to include your letters (RM etc.) after your name and a short biography that states, for example, that you 'also work as a midwife in the birth centre of a local maternity unit', although you should not give the name of the unit in which you work (see Boxes 5.1a, 5.1b and Activity 5.4).

As a doula or a midwife, you are also bound by certain restrictions on advertising, not least by the Advertising Standards Authority (ASA).[5] You are not permitted to make medical claims for the potential success of treatments, although you can use research to demonstrate that a treatment 'may' have a specific effect. For example, you could not claim that a treatment you provide to facilitate the onset of labour *will* be successful – here you might state that 'research shows that...' or that 'some maternity units now use...' to support your suggestion that the proposed treatment may work.

The ASA code applies to all forms of advertising in print, including leaflets, business cards, posters, circulars and other hard copy forms. It also applies to digital marketing such as websites, texts and SMS messages, faxes, social media advertising, blogs and advertorials (in which you write an 'article' about your business). There is a separate code for broadcast advertisements and different rules relating to premium-rate telephone services, advertisements in foreign media and some other forms of marketing.

Ensure that you proofread all advertising material thoroughly, using an English spell checker – spelling or typographical errors look very unprofessional. If you find it difficult, ask someone else to proofread your work before confirming it to your printers. For example, if you offer complementary therapies, ensure that the word 'complementary' is spelled with an 'e'! I once ordered some appointment cards to be printed and carefully proofread the Word file I sent to the printer, assuming that he would simply copy and paste my text into the

---

5   www.asa.org.uk

proposed format for printing. As a result, I was not vigilant enough when proofreading the draft, and when the final printed cards arrived, the word 'appointment' had only a single 'p'. Needless to say I was unable to use them and had to spend more money having them re-done.

Business cards

You should have some business cards prepared so that you can give them to prospective clients, business contacts and sources of possible referral. They are essential for any networking events you attend (see below). Whilst it is possible to obtain reasonably presentable business cards inexpensively, or even to design them online yourself, they can appear very amateurish and may detract from the image you are attempting to portray. Also, if you have used a graphic designer for your logo design it is better to have them sort out your business cards to ensure consistency, for example, the precise shade of colour you have chosen.

Business cards normally include your logo, your own name with any letters after your name (e.g., RM) and your title of choice (e.g., birth and postnatal doula; midwife acupuncturist). You should have all your contact details included – telephone number, website address, email address, social media addresses (Facebook, Twitter, Instagram, etc.). However, it is wise not to include your postal address if you work from home. You should also have a dedicated business email address; never use a jokey personal email address – plastered@company.co.uk is not an image you want to portray to your clients!

You may wish to use the reverse of the card to summarise in a single phrase what you offer (e.g., Support during and after pregnancy; Yoga for birth and babies), or use the space as an appointments card.

Writing your biography

Writing your biography for marketing purposes needs to sell you and your services and be written in a way that appeals to potential clients. You may want to include it on your advertising leaflets, your website and social media sites and any other ways in which you inform the public about your services. Summarising what you and your business offer is also a useful exercise when preparing for networking meetings, many of which require you to introduce yourself in under a minute.

Whilst you can draw on your *curriculum vitae*, if you have one, a biography is not simply a condensed summary of your career to date. You need to be able to show your passion, your enthusiasm and your personality, and it should be written in a way that is easily understood by the expectant parents who may be reading it. Experts recommend that a biography is written in the third person ('Jane is...') as this is considered more professional than the first person, although this may differ depending on your potential customers. On the other hand, some practitioners in the caring professions prefer to use the first person ('I am...') to give a more personal touch: this is entirely your decision. It can be useful to explore the biographies of other practitioners working in the maternity arena, such as pregnancy yoga teachers or maternity acupuncturists.

Your biography should be short and concise and between 200 and 500 words in length. Your name and what you do or the services you offer should be the very first things you write. Include a mention of your qualifications or additional training and your experience to date, but avoid using professional jargon and abbreviations. Include your most important achievements, certainly professional ones, but also perhaps personal accomplishments – you might include some personal information but take care that it will not compromise you or your family (for those working in the maternity field, this may be related to your personal experiences of childbirth). Some people include personal interests although this is not essential and may take up word space that could be better used for more professional information. You should conclude your biography either by highlighting your current work/passion or by summarising what you have to give to your potential clients. Boxes 5.1a and 5.1b give examples of a short biography, written in both the third and the first person, for use on printed leaflets and a website.

Box 5.1a: Example biography, written in the third person

Jane Smith BSc RM offers antenatal classes with a difference as well as one-to-one pregnancy and postnatal coaching and support. She began her career as a police officer, but following the births of her two children she wanted a change of direction and decided to train as an antenatal teacher and lactation consultant. Later she qualified as a midwife and she has seven years' experience of caring for women in pregnancy and during and after the birth; she continues to work part time as a midwife in a local maternity unit.

Jane was very fortunate to have both her children at home and has seen at first hand how having the same caring midwife throughout pregnancy can make so much difference to the birth experience. She is passionate about helping expectant parents to achieve the best birth possible through enhancing their understanding of pregnancy and the birth process.

Jane provides antenatal classes in [name of town] or one-to-one sessions in your own home if preferred, designed to empower you with the tools for a rewarding experience of birth and early parenthood. If you have specific issues you wish to discuss or are worried about your pregnancy or the birth of your baby, Jane has the time to listen and can suggest ways to help you feel more prepared. She also offers consultations to help you prepare for and establish breastfeeding as well as a 'birth after-thoughts' service to discuss any concerns about your labour.

Box 5.1b: Example biography, written in the first person

Hi, I'm Jane Smith BSc RM and I offer fabulous antenatal classes with a difference as well as one-to-one pregnancy and postnatal support. After the births of my two wonderful children (now aged 12 and 10) at home, I trained as an antenatal teacher and lactation consultant, then later decided to become a midwife. For the last seven years I've worked in several maternity units and as a community midwife and I continue to work part time in a local hospital.

I was very fortunate that both my children were born at home and I've seen at first hand how having the same caring midwife throughout pregnancy can make so much difference to the birth of your baby and the transition to becoming a parent. I'm passionate about helping you to achieve the best birth possible through an understanding of your pregnancy and the birth process.

I offer fabulous, fun birth preparation classes in [name of town] or one-to-one sessions in your own home if preferred. If you've got specific worries or just need someone to talk to about your pregnancy, I'm a good listener and can help you work things out. And afterwards, if you'd like help with breastfeeding problems or want to discuss any concerns about your labour, get in touch. I hope to meet you very soon.

✎ ACTIVITY 5.4: Writing your own biography

Now have a go at writing a biography for yourself. You may want to ask a colleague to help you with this – it is much easier to compliment someone else than to describe your own good points. When you have written your first draft, show it to several people whom you trust, and ask them to make suggestions for improvement.

Advertising leaflets

Even if you intend to do most of your marketing online, you will still need some hard copy leaflets to give to people you meet, prospective clients, professional contacts and networking associates. You may also want to put some in local GP surgeries and – if permissible – your local antenatal clinics, although these may need to be approved.

Advertising leaflets should be clear and concise and offer a brief summary of the main services you provide, a bit about you (this is a starting point to telling people about yourself but needs to be condensed to about 50 words) and your contact details. In addition, you may want to include a QR code, which is a machine-readable code consisting of an array of black and white squares that stores your website URL for reading by the camera on a smartphone.

It is wise not to include your prices – whilst you can change them easily on your website, you do not want to be left with loads of unused leaflets because you have increased your prices.

Using attention-grabbing headlines or rhetorical questions are useful tools to encourage people to look at your leaflets. Asking 'Pregnant?' rather than 'If you're pregnant…' is a better means of attracting potential clients. Being more specific can be even better: try something like 'Sick of being pregnant?' to advertise your treatments for nausea and vomiting. You should also try, with your headline question, to focus on the thing that really matters to your potential clients ('I feel ghastly with this morning sickness') and highlight the outcome (the end result) rather than the process so that women can see the benefit of using your services. In the example about nausea and vomiting treatments, you could ask, 'Have you thought about having acupuncture to ease that pregnancy sickness?' Using topical events or recent research findings can be helpful too – 'Research has shown that 72% of mums-to-be suffer sickness, with many struggling on their own to find a way to ease their symptoms.' (It is not necessary to provide the actual reference, but keep it in your records in case someone asks you for it – in this example the incidence is taken from Tan, Lowe and Henry 2017.)

You must be able to demonstrate your credibility, not just in general but if possible, specifically related to the issue. For example, 'Jane has treated over 300 women with pregnancy sickness and has

a 75% success rate in reducing symptoms in just two treatments.'
Include your USP – this might give the message that you are caring,
approachable and a good listener and that the services you provide are
intended to ensure the safety of mothers and babies. It also justifies
why women should come to you and reassures them that you may be
able to help them. It is good marketing practice to finish by asking
the reader (your potential client) to do something: 'Call now for an
appointment' or better still, 'Call 07956 123456 to speak to Jane and
book your appointment.'

Your leaflets should use as few words as possible to make your
point, leaving plenty of space – less is more. Wordy text is completely
counter-productive to your aim because people will be put off by
having to read so much to understand the message. The language must
be understandable and the colour and font must be striking but not
so unusual as to mask the message. Pale print on a dark background
is physically more difficult to read. Graphics are essential but use ones
for which you have paid, to avoid infringing copyright. The quality of
the finished leaflet will depend as much on the content as on how it is
presented, including the quality of the paper. Most leaflets are either
A5 size, and could have text or pictures on both sides, or commonly, a
single A4 sheet folded into three sections. This latter option provides
a front page, three separate pages inside to include information about
your services and about you, and a fifth page from the right-sided flap
folded inwards. The single back page should normally show just your
contact details.

Website

It is essential to have a professional website for your business and to
keep it updated and contemporary looking. Most expectant parents
will automatically turn to online searches to find the services they want
and often will not even consider accessing services from someone who
does not have a website. These days, not having a website is often seen
as amateurish, and this may cause people to think that your services
may also lack professionalism and credibility. If your potential clients
are online, then you need to be online too. Your website is not only a
means of drawing in new clients but also of providing information for

current and past customers – for example, where your clinic is based, your prices, new services that you may have added to your portfolio or just the facility for potential and current clients to ask a question via the 'Contact' button.

It is possible to design a simple website yourself but, as with business cards and advertising leaflets, this can lead to your site looking sub-standard and shoddy. If you have a friend or family member who is professionally skilled at designing websites (not just someone who likes doing it as a hobby), that may help, but be sure to treat the arrangement as a business contract, even if they are doing it for you free of charge. Give them a deadline by which you want the site completed, and ensure that they can source appropriate images and can organise web hosting for you. If you want to use a professional web designer, get at least three quotes and try to meet each one in person to see if the costings are acceptable and whether you can work with the company.

It is essential to research your market before designing the website because different demographics can influence the look and feel of the site, including font size and type and the language you need to use to have the greatest impact. It should not be too 'flashy' and must certainly not be too complex. We live in an age of immediacy, so remember: when expectant parents access your website, they probably already know what they want to find. It is said that if a visitor cannot find what they want within three seconds of landing on the home page, they are likely to give up and go elsewhere. Instilling in users of the site a sense of urgency to do something 'now' is also a good marketing tool and can be applied to other aspects of your business – indicating in some way, either on your website, your advertising literature or your responses to email or telephone enquiries, that you have limited availability for appointments makes people think that you must be very successful. For example, when a woman telephones you for an appointment, do not tell her that you cannot see her on Thursday because you are working in the maternity unit or are taking your children to the seaside; just tell her that that day is fully booked – you are not being untruthful, but she does not need to know that it is fully booked with NHS work or personal commitments!

The cost of designing and maintaining a website normally also includes the domain name (your web address such as www.your company.co.uk) and hosting, in other words the space on the internet for your site. Relatively inexpensive hosting is provided by companies such as GoDaddy[6] for a fairly nominal sum that is generally paid monthly. The web design may be free or chargeable according to the complexity of your site. You may need to pay extra for a dedicated email address associated with the web address, but this is a worthwhile expense because it will be similar to your web address, for example, www.maternitycare.co.uk and info@maternitycare.co.uk

Having your website professionally designed will mean that it has a contemporary feel and the web designer may be able to offer ideas for popular aspects such as the use of videos or interactive pages. The nature of communication in the 21st century is changing, with younger people often preferring to watch videos or look at pictures than to read large sections of text. Videos through YouTube will increase the traffic to your site – YouTube is owned by Google, so you gain higher rankings. A professionally designed site should also mean that your content is search engine optimised (SEO), which helps to place you prominently in searches undertaken by prospective clients. You should ensure that your website is responsive for mobile devices, ensuring that people using a mobile telephone or tablet can view the pages adequately.

As with your biography, your home page needs to state clearly who you are, what you do or the services you are offering and how to contact you. The site, and each of its pages, should be simple, clean and uncluttered, with a sense of identity and consistency between the pages. Visual images are essential, but do not use too many. You cannot simply take images from the internet as these may be copyrighted to the owner; you should use graphics that have been sourced from a company such as Shutterstock.[7] If you wish to use photographs of your past or current clients, you must have their written permission.

---

6   https://uk.godaddy.com
7   www.shutterstock.com

Case study: Samantha Jones BM Midwife; Diploma in Midwifery Complementary Therapies, Certificate in Midwifery Acupuncture

Natural Pregnancy (www.naturalpregnancy.wales), based in North Wales.

I was a senior student midwife whilst I was undertaking my aromatherapy diploma. Initially I commenced the course with a view to implementing aromatherapy in the NHS environment to enable equitable alternative service availability. However, it became apparent, quite quickly, that the NHS is not always open to alternative options for women, which made me very aware that standard policies and protocols may compromise individualised care. Women feel supressed in expressing their choices for their care and ultimately feel coerced into conforming to the NHS regime. I wanted to work in a way that enables me to deliver quality care and to meet the needs of my clients, building the mother–midwife relationship through continuity of carer, and providing support and choices to women to enhance their overall pregnancy and birth experience.

Having qualified as a midwife, I secured a part-time contract with my local trust and, at the same time, also completed the Expectancy Certificate in Midwifery Acupuncture. I set up my business in January 2018, having had my garage converted into a bespoke treatment room. I offer specialist advice and treatments using complementary therapies for women in the antenatal, intrapartum and postpartum periods. This includes acupuncture for pregnancy and postnatally, including nausea and vomiting, symphysis pubis discomfort and sciatica, reflex zone therapy (reflexology) and aromatherapy for relaxation and to treat pregnancy discomforts, support for recovery from birth and help with breastfeeding and specialist complementary therapy treatment for post-dates pregnancy.

I am very much still a start-up so I am constantly learning. I have identified my strengths and weaknesses. I have undertaken additional business-related courses to fill the gaps in my marketing knowledge whilst utilising my skills in office work to set up a good office environment and filing system. I envisage my turnover to be £10,000 this year; by next year I hope to be earning in the mid-£20,000s and by year 3 I aim to be bringing in £40,000.

Your greatest achievements? I am very humbled and touched by the lovely comments and reviews I have received even at this early stage of setting up the business. It is these sentiments that make me strive to ensure women know about my services and that, if they want them, they are available.

Your biggest mistake? I never thought it would be easy, but I didn't think I would face as many challenges in relation to complementary therapies as I have within the NHS setting. It is very important to ensure you have clear boundaries in respect of your private business and *any* NHS involvement. I thought I had mastered the concept and completed conflict of interest forms; I never discuss my private work in the NHS setting (especially not with the pregnant women), although I may discuss my private work in the staff room if asked by colleagues. I've learned that anything you write or post on social media will be dissected, so ensure there are no conflicts with groups you join or any statements you make. It is very challenging to stand up for your practice; however, I rise to this challenge in the knowledge I have been trained by the best. I follow my code of practice and have a duty to educate those not trained in complementary therapies as to the evidence-based benefits that provide real choices for women.

What is the best thing about working for yourself? Flexibility – I choose when I work so it fits around my family. I work from home so can put the dinner on, give a treatment, serve up dinner. Although I try to keep to time slots I do not feel pressured to do so and I provide time for women to communicate and discuss their needs, so there is less pressure as well!

What causes you most difficulty in running your own business? Marketing. It is a necessity but can become very time-consuming. As the business grows I expect that word of mouth and reputation of both myself and my treatments will sell the business 75 per cent, with around 1–2 hours of my time allocated to marketing each week. But this takes time.

What advice would you give to a midwife/doula who is just setting out in the commercial world? Do your homework, make sure there is a demand for your services in the area. Don't expect to be earning thousands in the first year, take your time and build quality – 'Rome wasn't built in a day'. Have guidelines and keep to them, especially for payments. This makes sure you practise safely and get paid in a timely manner.

Any other comments? I am so thankful that a talk on complementary therapies, which was arranged through our Midwifery Society when I was a student, resonated with me and sparked my passion for alternatives for women. My philosophy is underpinned by a desire for safe, women-centred care. Currently midwifery students are not trained in complementary therapies. Many midwives (unless self-funded) have little knowledge of the different therapies or how they interact with pregnancy anatomy and physiology. This can be unsafe as information is passed from midwife to woman in a Chinese whispers fashion. Higher education institutions and NHS trusts should consider practitioners as support mechanisms for good alternatives or enhancements to medical care, and embrace the knowledge and expertise to deliver care, as set out in documents such as *Midwifery 2020*.

Social media marketing

Social media are interactive online platforms that encourage communication between people and are about being *social*. Using social media as a means of marketing your business can be productive in that it can drive traffic to your main company website and increase your rankings. It helps to build your brand and is usually much less expensive than paying for formal advertising. It can help to boost your reputation but conversely, it can be damaging if negative comments are posted, either on your own site or on someone else's.

Remember, however, that social media marketing is not free because if you manage it yourself, it can be addictive and time-wasting – and time, including yours, is money. You need to manage it carefully and keep checking whether it is actually bringing you any business. It is better to schedule specific time in your diary to manage your social media sites and schedule your posts via a tool such as Hootsuite.[8] Avoid paying to advertise on social media unless you fully understand how it works.

Social networks include Facebook, the most popular site, as well as Google and for professional interaction, LinkedIn. Facebook and Google can be used to tell people about developments within

8   www.hootsuite.com

your company, such as new products or services, special offers and events you may be attending, for example, a local pregnancy fayre and exhibition. However, only about 30 per cent of your posts should be sales-focused. Including relevant news items, fascinating facts, celebrating special days such as Mother's Day or International Women's Day can all contribute to an interesting site that will draw people to it. Messaging platforms including Twitter, Snapchat and WhatsApp are suitable for short, sharp, instant messages, but the 'hard sell' approach is actively discouraged. These may be less appropriate for midwives and doulas in private practice, but it does depend how you use them and what you do. For example, I read once of a fisherman who had an unexpectedly good haul from the sea; he sent out Twitter messages to tell restaurateurs what he had available and where he was, and quickly sold all of his fish. Instagram is a site for sharing images and can be useful for companies in which images can help drive sales, such as the travel industry, but may not be so relevant to maternity-related services.

Social media management for your business is not something you do in your free time or when you remember to do it: it requires regular updating of your own content and responses to communications received, which can be a considerable time commitment. You may choose to pay someone to manage your social media content for you, but take care to brief them fully on how you wish your online presence to be seen. They must understand the basis of your business and the groups of potential clients you wish to engage in conversation. You do not want an inexperienced person who posts inappropriate items or who does not know where to source relevant news, research or other items you wish to include. Whoever manages your social media must be able to ensure that your search engine ranking will increase in order to expose you to as many people who may wish to use your services as possible.

Writing a blog

Blogging can be a useful marketing tool and, like your website, can boost your SEO, position your business as a leader in the field, even if it is just in your local area, connect to people wanting to use your services and increase your overall business income. Your blog also creates opportunities for sharing news about your company, your products and services and your reputation. Every time your blog is shared, liked, emailed or forwarded by some other media it spreads your reach far wider. A blog is usually hosted on your website and enables you to show the personal side of your business and of yourself, drawing out your personality – and remember, people buy people, particularly in the health and wellbeing sectors. It helps to build your brand identity and increase brand awareness. You can use your blog simply to encourage potential clients to buy from you, or you could use it to make money from advertising income and affiliate income through associations with other organisations. However, it can take some time to become an accomplished blog writer, so it may be wise to search the internet for tips on writing a successful blog or even consider attending a workshop to learn how to do it.

Exhibitions

You may have the opportunity to have a stand at a local exhibition or fayre for expectant parents and feel that this will reach a wide audience to which you can promote your services. Pregnancy and birth shows are big business and the exhibitions, even local ones, are likely to be well attended. It is certainly a way to create brand awareness in your area and, if you are exhibiting alongside other similar service providers, this will make you appear to be a credible business. Even if you do not actually sell much, there is a good chance that you will make some useful contacts through networking with other stallholders. If you do decide to have a stand, you will need public liability insurance and protection for your property (goods for sale, posters, banner stands, etc.) on-site. If you intend to offer short treatment sessions, such as hand massages, you must be in possession of specific insurance for performing at the exhibition.

However, be warned: exhibitions are expensive, because you have to pay for the table/stall space, spend time preparing well, have a banner stand made, produce sufficient hard copy literature to give out, use your valuable time, possibly pay others to help you on the day, and occasionally even pay for travel and accommodation if the exhibition is not in your local area. Exhibitions can be fun once you know what you are doing, but they are also stressful, incredibly exhausting and do not usually bring you the income you imagined – people often just take information away to peruse later rather than buying on the day. Furthermore, it is not merely a case of standing at the stall and thrusting leaflets into the hands of passers-by – you need very specific skills to turn both people expressing genuine interest in your services, as well as those just passing by your stand, into sales leads.

In the very early days of my business, when a team of clinical midwives worked with me, we decided to exhibit at two exhibitions – the Mother and Baby Show in Earls Court, West London, and a complementary therapies professional show in Docklands in East London. Unfortunately, I made a mistake about the dates and we discovered that both shows were being held on the same weekend. We were woefully under-prepared and had to buy two of everything in order to set up our stands in both places. I spent most of the weekend rushing backwards and forwards on the Underground between West and East London! I had also decided that we would need enough logo'd plastic bags in which to package any products we might sell. We had been told that we could expect around 5000 people to attend each show so I went ahead and ordered 10,000 plastic bags to be printed. Not only did we sell virtually nothing at either show, but I am also still using up the bags 15 years later!

Networking

Networking is a way of making connections and relationships with colleagues, both in professional (maternity-related) and in business services, and with potential clients. Joining a networking group, either in person or online, provides you with a forum to tell people about your business, what you offer and how you work. Networking groups enable you to meet people whose services you may wish to use, now or in the future, for example, accountants, lawyers, graphic designers, photographers, web developers or journalists. You can also share your own knowledge and expertise, and as you develop your confidence in running the business you will be able to help others.

Many business networking groups require their members to generate referrals at many or all of the meetings. These are often mixed groups with men and women from a wide range of small and medium-sized enterprises, and include large international organisations such as British Networking International (BNI)[9] or your local Chamber of Commerce.[10] Others serve more as support groups, particularly some of the women's-only groups, and tend to attract sole traders and micro-business owners, for example, the Athena Network.[11] It is important to try several groups as a visitor before committing to any particular one so that you can get a feel for the atmosphere and the ways they work. The Federation of Small Businesses[12] is not only a networking group but also an active campaigner on behalf of people working in small or micro-sized businesses. It also offers a wide range of benefits to members, including start-up information, legal and financial advice and referral sources.

Some networking groups charge an annual registration fee and a monthly meeting fee, which encourages members to commit fully to attending the meetings and to engage in other activities. These provide a learning forum as well as the opportunity to meet people, and many have regular seminars or talks from expert speakers, helping you to keep up-to-date with business matters, changes in the law or issues related to HM Revenue & Customs (HMRC). As with any marketing strategy, being visible by regularly meeting the same group helps to raise your personal profile so that other members remember the availability of your services and recognise your brand.

Other groups are free and often take the form of a coffee morning – you just turn up and buy a coffee, with no meeting fee to be paid, for example, LadiesWhoLatte.[13] This type can be attractive to people new to business as it does not cost a lot of money at a stage when you are spending cautiously. Free meetings also tend to have a rapid turnover of attendees, but this can work in your favour if you are targeting

9   www.bni.co.uk
10   www.britishchambers.org.uk
11   https://theathenanetwork.com
12   www.fsb.org.uk
13   www.ladieswholatte.com

women in your local area and want to meet as many as possible for minimal cost.

Some business groups act more as a problem-solving forum for members. I originally joined the Athena Network when I first started my company, primarily to meet other women in a semi-social setting as I had only recently moved to the area. This was instrumental in encouraging me to grow my business and I made contact with some wonderful colleagues, many of whom are now good friends. However, as I became more confident in running the business side of things, I found that I was no longer gaining as much as I had done previously – the monthly meetings had become a very expensive lunch occasion! I felt the need to be part of a group of close colleagues with whom I could share problems and consider new initiatives. As there was nothing like this in my area, I decided to set up something myself – and my newest venture, Expect Business Support, was born! Expect is a businesswomen's members-only problem-solving forum that meets monthly. We have 15 members and have come to know one another well so that we now feel comfortable in sharing sensitive or confidential issues that cannot always be discussed with day-to-day colleagues or staff.

In our field of work, it is also important to maintain contact with other midwives or doulas (or both), especially if you are no longer working in the NHS or have diversified your services beyond your original role. Keeping up-to-date with maternity issues, latest research and trends in standard maternity care is absolutely paramount, and you must remain aware of what is happening in education and practice within your profession. Sometimes it is good to know that you can ask a colleague amongst your networking contacts for advice about a particular client – or reciprocate if someone else has concerns. The commercial world can be a very lonely place at times and no more so than when you have completely removed yourself from the NHS system. Whilst you can ask any midwife friend or colleague for advice about clinical situations, you also need to discuss issues with others who appreciate the context in which you are working and the extra burdens you may face from being freelance. Joining your local Royal College of Midwives (RMC) meetings is one source of support for maternity matters, or you may prefer to contribute to an online forum.

Growing your business

It is essential to set short- and long-term plans for how you want your business to grow. Your business may evolve naturally as you add more services, or it may need to adapt to changes within the market. Since up to 80 per cent of businesses are thought to fail in the first 18 months, it is said that you are doing well if you can survive the first three years, and it is more likely that you will continue developing and growing. You need to take steps to ensure that your business will still be there in five or ten years' time (if that is what you want).

Initially, you will spend all your time on setting up the business and then providing your services, in other words, working 'in' the business, doing the day-to-day work. Later you need to work more 'on' the business, reflecting on income generation, reducing expenses, exploring different marketing strategies and evaluating what is working and what is not. Depending on your age and your family and personal circumstances, you may eventually also want to look at an exit strategy and consider succession planning if you want to keep the business going.

In business planning, it is common to use SMART goals – defining your goals by what is Specific, Measurable, Achievable, Relevant and Time-based. Having specific goals is the opposite of setting broad aims. These must be set in such a way that they can be measured objectively and the goal must be feasibly achieved within the time limit that you set. This format can be used from the outset, but is particularly useful once your business is established and evolving. You may have identified your broad aims but these can be clarified further by using the SMART goal format. Relevant growth pertains to income generation, increasing the number of clients or taking on more staff, rather than to operational (day-to-day) goals. You must also set a timely objective – a date by which you intend to achieve the goal you have identified. Box 5.2 gives an example of SMART goals that you may formulate at the start of setting up your business, using doula services as an example.

Box 5.2: An example of SMART goals at the beginning of your business

When you first think about starting a business, your broad aim may be 'I want to start a maternity-related business'. Using the SMART format, we can dissect this further:

- *Specific:* I want to provide birth and postnatal doula services.

- *Measurable:* I will be ready to take my first client within four weeks and I will aim to have a minimum of six clients in my first year.

- *Achievable:* I will advertise first on my website, Netmums and my new Facebook page, and I will make contact with local midwives, GPs and women's groups. I will also join some networking groups to promote my services.

- *Relevant:* Offering doula services will enable me to work with women in a way that I feel offers continuity, empowerment and advocacy for them to achieve the birth they want.

- *Time-based:* I will have my first client within four weeks of starting the business and will aim to have five more clients booked within the next six months.

When it comes to growing your business, you might say something like 'I want to be earning £40,000 by the end of year 3', so let us look now at how you can define SMART goals to help you, again using the doula example shown in Box 5.3. You can then try to work out your own goals in Activity 5.5.

Box 5.3: An example of SMART goals at the beginning of your business

- *Specific:* I will acquire 15 clients a year for birth and/or postnatal services by the end of year 2.

- *Measurable:* I will measure my progress by how many new clients I take on each month and maintaining a comprehensive database.

- *Achievable:* I will ask current clients for referrals, launch an active social media marketing campaign, contact past clients for referrals, liaise with antenatal class facilitators, advertise in the local NCT magazine and network with three different sources of people in the 20–45 age group.

> • *Relevant:* Adding new clients to my business will allow me to grow my business and increase my income.
>
> • *Time-based:* I will have five new clients within the next four months.

✎ ACTIVITY 5.5: Defining your own SMART goals to grow your business

– Think back to the main reasons why you chose to go into private practice/set up your own business (you may want to refer back to the activities in Chapters 1 and 2 for this).

– What did you feel, at that time, were your ultimate goals for your business?

– Have your long-term goals changed since starting the business? If so, what do you feel, in broad terms, are your new medium- to long-term goals?

– Write a broad goal: 'I want to…'

- Now, using the SMART format, re-write your broad aim, breaking it down into a one-year and a five-year goal:

  - Specific:

  - Measurable:

  - Achievable:

  - Relevant:

–   Time-based:

There are several small ways in which you can grow your business. At a basic level, in order to increase the transfer of income into your account, you could invoice clients prior to appointments and ask for payment within 7 days rather than 30. You could examine all your expenditure and see how you could reduce it by, say, 20 per cent. You could evaluate your marketing strategies and try to expand the listings and links for your online presence.

You could outsource – this means paying someone to do some of the work that takes up your time or that you do not like doing or do not do well. This might be something like getting a cleaner if you work from home or consulting a professional to take on your regular social media posts. If you have staff, learn to delegate instead of trying to do everything yourself (a common problem in small businesses, not just on financial grounds but by virtue of the fact that small business owners generally like to be in control).

You could simplify the services you offer to focus on a niche market, perhaps by offering high-end packages. A package is not giving discounts such as 'six for the price of five' but is based on providing value for money for the desired outcome – for example, 'I will help to prepare you for the birth of your baby and becoming a parent.' Packages are generally costed at *more* than the sum of their component parts because they include intangible aspects that cannot be costed, such as 'continuity of carer' or 'unlimited telephone access to ask me any questions you may have' (although I suggest you prohibit calls in the middle of the night, unless a woman has gone into labour!).

Other ways to increase your income include adding new services or selling products, selling more to your existing clients and taking on new clients who may want services you have not offered before. You could also widen your access by looking at online services, for example, Skype-type consultations for aspects that do not require you to be physically with the woman. Indirect marketing such as offering to speak at events, writing a blog or compiling a newsletter and undertaking some related charitable work may all bring in extra business. Having a good after-sales strategy can also help – sending a card on the birth of the baby, or a thank you card for the client's business will help too, and asking for evaluations from clients, using one or two good ones (with permission) for testimonials on your website or Facebook page, is also an excellent way of convincing others to use your services.

Case study: Amanda Redford BSc (Hons) Midwifery, BSc (Hons) Complementary Medicine

Acupuncturist and clinical complementary healthcare specialist for pregnancy, fertility and women's health (www.amandaredford.com or www.facebook.com/AmandaRedfordHolistic), based in Staffordshire in the Midlands.

After qualifying as a midwife, I wanted to set up a complementary therapy service in the NHS, but this was not to be. Having trained in acupuncture, reflexology, aromatherapy, massage and specialist therapies for fertility treatment, I was aware that more and more pregnant women wanted to use complementary therapies, so I decided to set up in private practice in 2010 and I have never looked back. I started working from home, then rented my own premises. I now also work in a high-quality professional health and wellbeing clinic for women's health. I funded the start-up of the business myself and as I was running it part time, this worked for me. Currently my income from private work is below £20,000, but I hope to expand my business and make it a full-time practice. I currently work part time as an NHS research midwife and have contributed to studies on acupuncture for back pain in pregnancy as well as many other obstetric and gynaecology trials.

Your greatest achievements? Feeling a sense of making a real difference to the women I see, being recognised and respected for what I do. The communication I have with women, the ongoing relationships with clients and the wonderful testimonials I have received make me feel honoured to be able to offer women services I truly believe in.

How has your business evolved since you first started? I initially trained in several therapies and offered services on a general basis, but over the years my practice has become specialised in the areas I am most passionate about – pregnancy, women's health and fertility. This has given me more confidence and allowed me the freedom to study at a deeper level, giving me an in-depth knowledge and a wealth of experience in order to offer a high-quality service.

What is the best thing about working for yourself? Being in control of everything in relation to work–life balance; planning my own hours and time off. Freedom to explore and enjoy new ideas. Developing my skills and knowledge within a specialised area of interest.

What causes you most difficulty in running your own business? Combining private work with NHS work – you have to be careful about conflicts of interest and energy levels can be affected when juggling several part-time jobs, particularly when seeing private clients in the evening following a full working day. Initially I struggled with marketing my practice due to a lack of social media presence and not targeting specific areas to reach appropriate audiences.

What advice would you give to a midwife/doula who is just setting out in the commercial world? Understand the market you wish to be working in: do your research, check out the local competition and what is on offer. Be prepared to invest a lot of hard work and time into your business – many hours will be unpaid. Ensure that your products/services are the best and there is a demand for them. Network with as many people/places/groups as you can for support, development and help to build your business. Regular continuing professional development is equally important. Never become complacent. Believe in yourself and your products/services and be 100 per cent confident. Do not under-value yourself. Be passionate. Do what you love and love what you do. And always remember to look after yourself.

Conclusion

In this book I have tried to give you some tips for making your new maternity-related business a success. I have, I hope, covered some of the many business-related issues that you need to consider and shared some of my own experiences and mistakes so that you can avoid similar problems. As a midwife or doula there is so much to learn about setting up and running a business, so do not think that this book has all the answers.

Using the services of a business coach or consultant can be helpful once you have started trading. A business coach is a little like a counsellor, facilitating you to work out for yourself what needs to be done to grow your business and to make it successful. A business coach challenges your thinking, your goals and your willingness to grow, and provides you with both the practical and mental tools needed to steer you towards your ultimate goal. They challenge you to think outside your comfort zone in order to help you to make your ideas a reality and to be accountable for the way your business evolves. You have the personal attention of someone who is an expert in business principles and who, with your help, comes to know your business almost as well as you. This increases your confidence and pushes you further than you may have been able to go on your own.

I have been mentoring midwives wanting to set up in their own practice for some years now, and I love hearing their ideas and helping them to achieve their dreams. Although you do not have to have a business coach from your own professional field, I do feel that it helps because you do not have to start at the beginning as you would with a coach who knows nothing about the maternity arena and the culture in which we work. Contact me at info@expectancy.co.uk for more information.

To reiterate what I said at the beginning of this book, running a business is a marathon, not a sprint. This is only the beginning of your journey towards your new business and the rest is up to you. Good luck!

Glossary

Cash flow	The amount of money that a company receives or pays out in expenses
Companies House	UK governmental executive agency that acts as the registrar of companies, under the remit of the Department for Business, Energy and Industrial Strategy
Company director	Owner of a limited company who owns at least one share in the business and who is responsible for aspects of the day-to-day management and/or financial management of the business
Company secretary	Official of a limited company who deals with financial and legal issues; a limited company is required to appoint a company secretary, who may also be one of the directors
Corporation Tax	Tax payable on profits from a limited company and certain other organisations – currently 19%
Her Majesty's Revenue & Customs (HMRC)	UK government non-ministerial department responsible for collection of taxes, social support payments and certain regulatory processes
Limited company	Private company, registered with Companies House, the owners of which are protected from personal bankruptcy through limited liability
Limited liability	The legal protection afforded to shareholders in a limited company – the obligation of individual shareholders for the debts of the company are limited to the value of their shares
National Insurance	Percentage of salary paid to the government in order to be eligible for state pension and other benefits

P11D	Statutory form submitted to HMRC detailing cash value of benefits and expenses paid to company directors
P45	Document provided by employer on leaving their employment, detailing income and tax paid; must be retained for at least five years
P60	Form provided annually by an employer stating how much taxable income was earned by the individual and how much tax has been paid; must be retained for at least five years
Partnership	Association of two or more people engaged in a for-profit business; may be general or limited partnership
Personal professional indemnity insurance	Insurance to cover the costs of law suits and expenses in defending a claim for negligence and compensation payable to the client in the event of being found liable; a legal requirement of all healthcare practitioners
Product liability insurance	Insurance to cover the costs of legal expenses and compensation claims if a company is found liable for injury or damage caused by products sold by or supplied through the business
Public liability insurance	Insurance to cover the legal costs and compensation claims payable by a company if someone is injured or their property is damaged whilst at your business premises or if you work in their home, office or business property
Sole trader	An exclusive owner of a business, entitled to keep all profits (after tax) but also liable for all losses
Turnover	The amount of money (income) taken by a business in any given period
Value Added Tax (VAT)	Tax payable on the purchase of products, most business transactions and goods from certain services. Some products are excluded; others have a reduced rate. Businesses must register for VAT once the income reaches a specified amount – currently 20% if the total income is over £83,000 in any one year

References and Useful Resources

Adams, J., Steel, A., Frawley, J., Broom, A. and Sibbritt, D. (2017) 'Substantial out-of-pocket expenditure on maternity care practitioner consultations and treatments during pregnancy: Estimates from a nationally-representative sample of pregnant women in Australia.' *BMC Pregnancy Childbirth 17*(1), 114.

Anadaciva, S. (2017) 'NHS myth-busters.' London: The King's Fund, 20 November Available at www.kingsfund.org.uk/publications/nhs-myth-busters

ATC (Aromatherapy Trade Council) (2011) 'Selling & Manufacturing Aromatherapy Products.' 4 August. Available at www.a-t-c.org.uk/frequently-asked-questions/general-faqs

Bastard, J. and Tiran, D. (2009) 'Aromatherapy and massage for antenatal anxiety, its effect on the fetus.' *Complementary Therapies in Clinical Practice 15*(4), 48–54.

BBC News (2018) 'NHS: Over 3,000 more midwifery training places offered.' Available at www.bbc.co.uk/news/health-43529877

Bohren, M.A., Hofmeyr, G., Sakala, C., Fukuzawa, R.K. and Cuthbert, A. (2017) 'Continuous support for women during childbirth.' *Cochrane Review.* Available at www.cochrane.org/CD003766/PREG_continuous-support-women-during-childbirth

Campbell, D. and Duncan, P. (2016) 'Is "incessant increase" in caesarean births putting first-time mothers' health at risk?' *The Guardian*, 31 January. Available at www.theguardian.com/society/2016/jan/31/caesarean-health-risks-c-section-first-time-mothers

DH (Department of Health) (1970) *The Peel Report.* London: HMSO.

DH (1993) *Changing Childbirth. Report of the Expert Maternity Group.* London: HMSO.

Fearn, H. (2015) 'Pregnant women employ "doulas" for support during labour as NHS cuts hit.' *The Independent Online*, 20 April. Available at www.independent. co.uk/life-style/health-and-families/health-news/pregnant-women-employ-doulas-for-support-during-labour-as-nhs-cuts-hit-10190834.html

Gbadamosi, N. (2015) 'Why the NHS must replicate retail.' *Health Services Journal*, 6 November. Available at www.hsj.co.uk/why-the-nhs-must-replicate-retail/5091475.article

Gerada, C. (2014) 'Something is profoundly wrong with the NHS today.' *BMJ Careers*, 16 June. Available at http://careers.bmj.com/careers/advice/view-article.html?id=20018022

King's Fund, The (2015) 'Is the NHS being privatised?' Available at www. kingsfund.org.uk/projects/verdict/nhs-being-privatised

Merrifield, N. (2017) 'Ageing midwifery workforce on "cliff edge" warns RCM.' *Nursing Times*, 7 February. Available at www.nursingtimes.net/ news/workforce/ageing-uk-midwife-workforce-on-cliff-edge-warns-rcm/7015420.article

Midwifery 2020 (2010) *Midwifery 2020: Delivering Expectations* [ebook]. London: Department of Health. Available at https://www.gov.uk/government/ uploads/system/uploads/attachment_data/file/216029/dh_119470.pdf

Moore, A. (2017) 'How codes are raising the bar.' *Health Services Journal*, 7 June, 10–13.

MSAC (Maternity Services Advisory Committee) (1982) *Maternity Care in Action, Part I – Antenatal Care. First Report of the Maternity Services Advisory Committee.* London: HMSO.

MSAC (1984) *Maternity Care in Action, Part II – Care During Childbirth (Intrapartum Care). Second Report of the Maternity Services Advisory Committee to the Secretaries of State for Social Services and for Wales.* London: HMSO.

MSAC (1985) *Maternity Care in Action, Part III – Care of the Mother and Baby (Postpartum Care). Third Report of the Maternity Services Advisory Committee to the Secretaries of State for Social Services and for Wales.* London: HMSO.

Mulroy, Z. (2017) 'This is how much it could cost you to give birth without our NHS.' *Daily Mirror*, 7 June. Available at www.mirror.co.uk/news/politics/ privatised-nhs-cost-of-childbirth-10577787

National Maternity Review (2016) *Better Births: Improving Outcomes in Maternity Services in England.* Available at www.england.nhs.uk/wp-content/uploads/ 2016/02/national-maternity-review-report.pdf

NMC (Nursing and Midwifery Council) (2015) *The Code: Professional Standards of Practice and Behaviour for Nurses and Midwives.* Available at www.nmc.org.uk/ standards/code/read-the-code-online

NMC (2017) *Guidance on Using Social Media Responsibly*. Available at www.nmc.org.uk/globalassets/sitedocuments/nmc-publications/social-media-guidance.pdf

ONS (Office for National Statistics) (2016) 'Births in England and Wales: 2016.' Available at www.ons.gov.uk/peoplepopulationandcommunity/birthsdeaths andmarriages/livebirths/bulletins/birthsummarytablesenglandandwales/2016

Patients4NHS (2018) 'Private companies' involvement in the NHS.' Available at www.patients4nhs.org.uk/private-companies-involvement-in-the-nhs

Schwab, W., Marth, C. and Bergant, A.M. (2012) 'Post-traumatic stress disorder post partum: The impact of birth on the prevalence of post-traumatic stress disorder (PTSD) in multiparous women.' *Geburtshilfe Frauenheilkd 72*(1), 56–63.

Sweet, B. and Tiran, D. (1990) 'Complementary Therapies in Pregnancy and Birth.' In B. Sweet and D. Tiran (eds), *Mayes' Midwifery* (11th edn). Edinburgh: Bailliere Tindall.

Tan, A., Lowe, S. and Henry, A. (2017) 'Nausea and vomiting of pregnancy: Effects on quality of life and day-to-day function.' *Australian and New Zealand Journal of Ostetrics and Gynaecology 58*(3), 278–290.

Tiran, D. (2004) *Nausea and Vomiting in Pregnancy: An Integrated Approach*. Edinburgh: Elsevier.

Tiran, D. (2014) *Maternity Complementary Therapies: Professional Code of Practice*. Available at http://expectancy.co.uk/files/shop/downloads/37/PROFESSIONAL%20CODE%20OF%20PRACTICE.pdf

Tiran (2017) *Bailliere's Midwives' Dictionary*. Edinburgh: Elsevier.

Tiran, D. (2018) *Complementary Therapies in Maternity Care: An Evidence-Based Approach*. London: Singing Dragon.

Vian, T., White, E.E., Biemba, G., Mataka, K. and Scott, N. (2017) 'Willingness to pay for a maternity waiting home stay in Zambia.' *Journal of Midwifery & Women's Health 62*(2), 155–162.

Useful resources

British Chambers of Commerce: www.britishchambers.org.uk

Business Is Great: www.greatbusiness.gov.uk

Companies House: www.gov.uk/government/organisations/companies-house

Federation of Small Businesses: www.fsb.org.uk

Her Majesty's Revenue & Customs (HMRC): www.gov.uk/government/organisations/hm-revenue-customs

HMRC business support: www.gov.uk/business-support-helpline

Index

By the same author

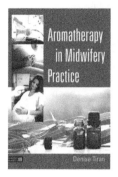

Aromatherapy in Midwifery Practice
Denise Tiran

Paperback: £22.99 / $39.95
ISBN: 978 1 84819 288 1
eISBN: 978 0 85701 235 7
232 pages

Aromatherapy is increasingly incorporated into midwifery practice, particularly in midwife-led units. It is the most commonly used therapy by midwives and birthing practitioners but access to up-to-date safety information is limited. Almost 90% of women may be using complementary therapies during pregnancy and birth and so it is very important that midwives are aware of safe and appropriate use based on contemporary evidence. This book covers safety, effectiveness, evidence, benefits and risks, and legal, ethical and professional issues related to incorporating aromatherapy into maternity care. Useful charts and tables are included for quick reference in clinical practice, making this is the ultimate handbook for using aromatherapy in midwifery practice.

The scientific basis behind aromatherapy, including relevant anatomy and physiology, chemistry and pharmacology are covered, as well as a critical appraisal of the contemporary research evidence supporting the use of aromatherapy in maternity care. Essential oil profiles of the oils that can be safely used in pregnancy, birth and postnatally are also included.

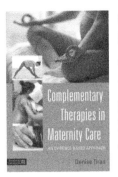

Complementary Therapies in
Maternity Care
An Evidence-Based Approach
Denise Tiran

Paperback: £24.99 / $39.95
ISBN: 978 1 84819 328 4
eISBN: 978 0 85701 284 5
352 pages

The complete textbook on complementary therapies in maternity care, this book addresses how midwives and other birth professionals can use or advise on complementary therapies for pregnant, labouring and new mothers.

Almost 90% of women may be using complementary therapies during pregnancy and birth, and increasingly midwives and doulas incorporate therapies into their care of women, so it is vital that they and other professionals in the maternity care field are aware of safe and appropriate use based on contemporary evidence. Therapies covered include acupuncture, herbal medicine, homeopathy, aromatherapy, reflexology, yoga, massage and hypnosis.

This complete guide to complementary therapies in pregnancy and childbirth covers safety, effectiveness, evidence, benefits and risks, legal, ethical and professional issues based on accurate and up-to-date research.

CPI Antony Rowe
Eastbourne, UK
October 19, 2023